60 tips

headaches

Marie Borrel

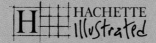
HACHETTE Illustrated

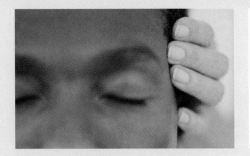
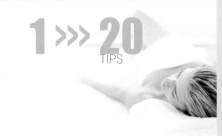

TIPS

contents

introduction 4
how to use this book 7
assessing your headache 8

useful addresses 124
index 125
acknowledgements 126

Note: The information and recommendations given in this book are not intended to be a substitute for medical advice. Consult your doctor before acting on any recommendations given in this book. The authors and publisher disclaim any liability, loss, injury or damage incurred as a consequence, directly or indirectly, of the use and application of the contents of this book.

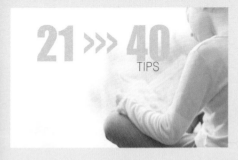

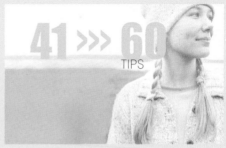

21 >>> 40
TIPS

41 >>> 60
TIPS

introduction

Headaches are a real pain!

A huge proportion of people – perhaps as many as one in ten – suffer from headaches and the great majority of them are women.

'Piercing ... insidious ... burning ... throbbing ... it strikes when you least expect it' – are just some of the descriptions given by migraine sufferers. Pain grips your skull, extends across your forehead and grinds into your temples. You feel grim. The pain continues remorselessly, or bright lights start to flash before your eyes. Whatever form it takes, the condition can become a real handicap, especially if attacks occur more and more often. The general medical term for all these pains is cephalalgia and they can arise from pain receptors in the head and neck. Although there are many serious causes of headaches, such as acute meningitis or cerebral haemorrhage, and less serious causes like acute sinusitis or dental problems, the vast majority of people with recurrent headaches have a disorder that, although uncomfortable, has no major implications for their health.

The most common cause of chronic headache, i.e., headaches on a daily basis or several times a week over a period of many months or years, is tension headache. The sufferer complains of a tight band around the head, or throbbing or bursting pains. There is no problem with vision and symptoms are often associated with stress or depression. Neurologists usually make the diagnosis by simply talking to the patient about their symptoms, and blood tests or brain scans are only carried out if there is something unusual in the medical history.

Migraine, as its classical Greek origin ('hemikrania') indicates, usually affects only one half of the head, and is a form of recurrent headache associated with visual disturbance and symptoms such as vomiting. Headaches come in bouts lasting hours or days with periods of complete freedom between episodes. Migraine often runs in families and there are often recognized triggers such as missing meals, foods like red wine or cheese, or menstruation.

These headaches are very common and often overlap. They may also develop into a form of daily headache due to over-consumption of painkillers.

Not all headaches are alike

As far as doctors are concerned, headaches are a real pain! The form they take, their causes and the factors that trigger an attack differ from person to person. Despite this diversity, the following categories of migraine headaches are used:

'Common' migraines attack without warning or apparent reason. The pain, which is sharp and throbbing, often begins first thing in the morning. It is felt in the fore-head, usually on one side only, and sometimes at the back of the eyes or in the temples, and is accompanied by nausea, sometimes even vomiting, constipation or diarrhoea, and dizziness. The sufferer is pale, tired and can hardly get up to start the day. About 70% of migraine headaches fall into this category.

'Classical' migraines are preceded by visual symptoms such as flashing lights, black spots and shining or coloured blotches. Sometimes there is abnormal sen-sitivity to sound and the patient feels nauseous and may vomit. These symptoms are followed by tingling sensations on the palms of the hands or around the mouth. This is the beginning of the attack. Sufferers are often irritable and prefer to lie in a darkened room and try to sleep, which relieves the headaches. These headaches, although just as disturbing as the first kind, do not arrive without warning, enabling the sufferer to try to prevent the pain from occurring.

The mechanism of migraine is unknown but it may be caused by changes in the activity of the trigeminal nerve, which supplies the face. Levels of neurotransmitters such as serotonin alter, triggering dilation of the large blood vessels in the meninges and the surface of the brain, leading to a throbbing headache. There is a strong genetic factor and a series of recognized triggers in people with a tendency to develop migraine. You run a 60% risk of suffering from headaches if one of your parents is subject to them and an 80% risk if both of them suffer. It's unfair but that's just the way it is. Susceptibility generally becomes apparent during childhood or adolescence.

Psychological factors, such as strong emotion or stress, can play a crucial role in triggering headaches, as sufferers know only too well. Irritation, suppressed anger and overtiredness can all cause an attack, if you're liable to them. Periods of feverish agitation followed by moods of despondency also spell trouble for those subject to headaches.

Hormones can be to blame

The fact that many more women than men suffer from headaches is undoubtedly due to hormonal differences. The hormonal life of a man can be seen as moving smoothly forward in a straight line, whereas that of a woman is marked by constant repetitions, waves and cycles, so there are many more factors that can cause an hormonal imbalance; migraine may start around puberty, can vary with the menstrual cycle and may be worsened by the contraceptive pill. A reduction in blood sugar level caused by missing meals can prompt violent headaches, as sufferers know to their cost, as can some of the things we eat and drink, such as chocolate, eggs, fats and alcohol. Skipping breakfast and snacking on a cheese sandwich or chocolate bar at lunchtime may trigger migraine in those who are susceptible.

A silver lining

The fact that there are so many different causes has its positive side, because it means there are many lifestyle or natural treatments for headaches: dietary changes, herbal or Chinese medicine, exercise, water cures, massage and psychotherapy are all ways of dealing with the problem. And if none of these works, then modern medicine does have some effective options.

However, first and foremost, you need to recognize the causes of your pain and the times when it is likely to strike. Once the nature of the problem is fully understood, it becomes much easier to control and remedy.

how to use this book

● ● ● FOR YOUR GUIDANCE

> **A symbol at the bottom of each page will help you to identify the natural solutions available:**

Herbal medicine, aromatherapy, homeopathy, Dr Bach's flower remedies – how natural medicine can help.

Simple exercises – preventing problems by strengthening your body.

Massage and manipulation – how they help to promote well-being.

Healthy eating – all you need to know about the contribution it makes.

Practical tips for your daily life – so that you can prevent instead of having to cure.

Psychology, relaxation, Zen – advice to help you be at peace with yourself and regain serenity..

> **A complete programme that will solve all your health problems. Try it!**

This book offers a made-to-measure programme, which will enable you to deal with your own particular problem. It is organized into four sections:

• **A questionnaire** to help you to assess the extent of your problem.
• **The first 20 tips** that will show you how to change your daily life in order to prevent problems and maintain health and fitness.
• **20 slightly more radical tips** that will develop the subject and enable you to cope when problems occur.
• **The final 20 tips** which are intended for more serious cases, when preventative measures and attempted solutions have not worked.

At the end of each section someone with the same problem as you shares his or her experiences.

You can go methodically through the book from tip 1 to 60 putting each piece of advice into practice. Alternatively, you can pick out the recommendations which appear to be best suited to your particular case, or those which fit most easily into your daily routine. Or, finally, you can choose to follow the instructions according to whether you wish to prevent stress problems occurring or cure ones that already exist.

Assessing your headache

Read the following statements and tick box **A** if you rarely suffer from these problems, box **B** if you often suffer from them and box **C** if you suffer from them all the time.

A	B	C	
A	B	C	You sleep badly and wake up feeling tired.
A	B	C	You suffer with back problems.
A	B	C	You have no regular eating pattern.
A	B	C	You use stimulants like tobacco, alcohol, coffee.
A	B	C	Your attacks always start at the same time of day.

A	B	C	
A	B	C	Your headaches occur when the rhythm of life changes, such as at holiday times.
A	B	C	Others in your family suffer from headaches.
A	B	C	You tend to lead a very stressful life.
A	B	C	Certain foods cause you headaches.
A	B	C	Your headaches can last for several days.

If you have ticked mostly **A**s, ` Tips **1** to **20** will suit you best. .

If you have ticked mostly **B**s, turn directly to Tips **21** to **40**.

If you have ticked mostly **C**s, go immediately to Tips **41** to **60**. It's time to take action!

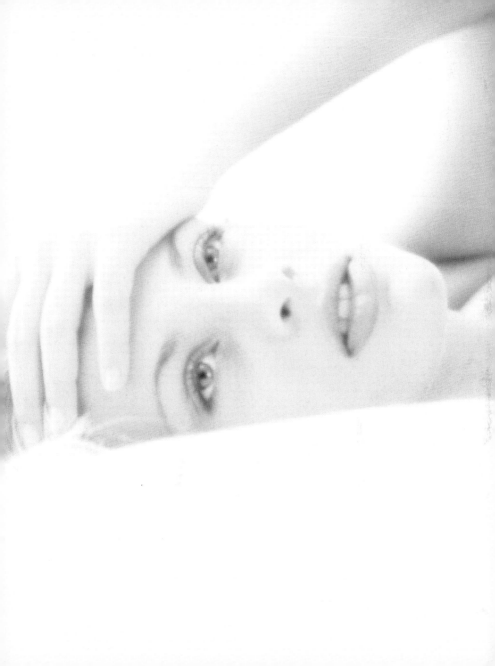

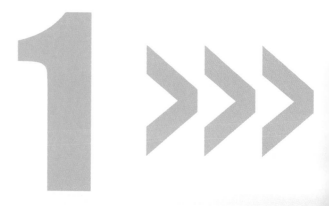

The pain starts up and steadily gets worse. Sometimes it just won't go away. Whether headaches affect your eyes, the back of your head, your temples or one side of your head (true migraines, technically speaking), they can be unbearable and make your social and family life hard to handle.

If this doesn't happen very often, there are some simple ways of avoiding attacks or dealing quickly with them when they do strike.

Here are 20 tips for a healthy lifestyle, to tackle the most important matter first.

20
TIPS

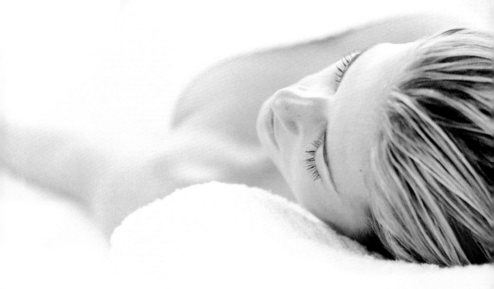

01

Headaches are sometimes caused by what you eat or drink: dairy products, chocolates or eggs, for instance. This is your body's way of protesting against what you are giving it. Listen to your body and learn to understand what it's saying. It will thank you for it.

identify headache-inducing foods

Food intolerance

About 20% of headaches are caused by food and drinks such as chocolate, cheese and other dairy products, wine and other forms of alcohol, caffeine, fermented foods like pickled herring, citrus fruits and sometimes by other products that are normally harmless.

Although it remains as yet scientifically unproven, food intolerance is something with which many headache sufferers are

●●● D'ID YOU KNOW?

> Some people are particularly sensitive to monosodium glutamate (MSG). This substance, found in many Chinese and Japanese dishes, is used as a flavour enhancer.

> This means it is used to improve the taste of food, rather like salt in western cookery. It can cause severe migraine attacks in some people.

very familiar. If you know which food bring on your attacks, the solution is simple: don't eat them. If not, keep a detailed note of your reactions for several weeks and perhaps you'll discover the guilty product.

Looking for the guilty product

If you suspect that something in your normal diet is giving you headaches, avoid it completely for at least a month. In this way, you'll be able to check if your suspicions are justified.

If you have no particular suspicions, keep a diary: in one column note down everything you eat and drink and in another, everything concerning the attacks, such as dates and intensity. You should be able to easily see any connections, and then you can double-check your findings.

Make sure you eliminate from your diet only one food at a time. This is the only way to monitor the effects of each one.

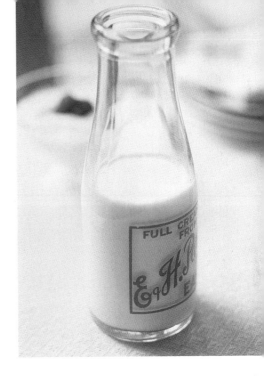

> If you are one of these, avoid Chinese and Japanese restaurants and look carefully at food labels when out shopping. The food industry often uses MSG as a flavouring in pre-cooked dishes.

    KEY FACTS

* Check out certain foods and drinks carefully: chocolate, cheese and dairy products, wine, alcohol, citrus fruits and processed meats.

* Don't consume anything you're not sure about.

* Keep a diary to check whether your headaches are caused by something you eat or drink.

02

change the way you eat

If you want to get rid of your headaches, now's the time to change what you eat. Learn to eat a healthier, fresher, more varied diet and also avoid missing meals; eat regularly. You'll be less tired, less stressed and what's more, less liable to headaches.

Freshness and variety are the key

To stay healthy, with plenty of mental and physical energy, you need to eat healthily. Headaches are often triggered and made worse by nervous tension caused by tiredness and stress. If your body lacks vitamins and minerals, it will cope less well with tension. A balanced diet may not have a direct effect on headaches but it's always best to ensure that all the cards are stacked in your favour. It's time

● ● ● DID YOU KNOW?

> If you're worried about calculating the right proportions, just use the 4–2–1 rule.

> Try to ensure that your daily intake contains 4 parts carbohydrates (cereals, fruit and vegetables), 2 parts proteins (meat, fish, eggs) and 1 part lipids (fats).

to get down to fundamentals and change what you eat. The basic rules of healthy eating are simple: fresh food and variety. Even if you can't eat some foods, there's still an enormous range available to you. Try to eat good-quality produce, preferably organic.

A little bit of everything

• Firstly, fruit and vegetables (at least three portions per meal). They contain vitamins and minerals as well as water, sugar and fibre. Half of your intake should be eaten raw, as cooking destroys some essential vitamins.
• Then cereals: they provide energy and fibre and stop you from feeling hungry.
• Don't forget proteins: lean meat, fish and eggs (for those who can tolerate them). They build muscle.
• The fats: these should be vegetable fats and preferably uncooked (see p. 22).
• Finally, avoid white sugar (see p. 16).

> Beware however of hidden elements, such as the fat in meat and the sugar in confectionery and fizzy drinks.

A little tip: if you want to make sure you're not lacking any vitamins or minerals, regularly vary the colour (red, yellow, green, purple) of the fruit and vegetables you eat. Their colours are due to their chemical constituents, including vitamins and minerals. Vary the colours and you vary the nutrients.

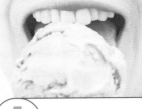

KEY FACTS

* Healthy eating means more physical and mental energy. If you are less tired, you will have less stress and fewer headaches.

* Eat a little of everything but nothing to excess. Make sure your food is fresh, varied and of good quality.

* Don't forget organic food.

03

Some headaches occur because the body has difficulty dealing with sugar. A sudden fall in the blood sugar level is a common cause of headaches. Learn to choose 'good' sugars and avoid 'bad' ones. The main enemy is white sugar.

shun white sugar

Rapid- and slow-release sugars

There are several kinds of sugar. Some of them (complex carbohydrates) are composed of long chains of sugar molecules joined together, whilst others (simple sugars) are made up of only two molecules of sugar. The former, also known as slow-release sugars, need to be broken down in the stomach before passing into the bloodstream. The second kind, rapid-release sugars, pass much more quickly into the bloodstream. The sugars are then distributed around the body's cells by the blood. Insulin, produced by the pancreas, regulates the blood sugar level: if the pancreas does not make enough insulin for the body's needs, then the blood sugars will be high – which is what happens in diabetes; too much insulin and the blood sugars will be too low, leading to hypoglycaemia.

Complex sugars are found in foods such as cereals, pasta and bread. Fruit (fructose) and refined products such as chocolate, jam, sweets, fizzy drinks and of course white sugar (glucose) are all sources of simple sugars.

Too much or too little

When simple glucose rushes into the bloodstream (hyperglycaemia), the body calls on the pancreas to secrete a large amount of insulin so that the glucose can be put into storage in the liver, muscles and fat. The pancreas responds and the

blood sugar level falls. However, the reduction is so rapid in some people that their blood sugar level falls too low. This is hypoglycaemia, causing fatigue, dizziness and, above all, headaches.

The immediate solution is to eat a lump of white sugar. This works in the short term but eventually the situation will get worse. Those who are susceptible to hypoglycaemia should gradually wean themselves off refined sugar in order to control their blood sugar levels. This should be done by gradually replacing rapid-release sugars with fruit and a regular intake of slow-release sugars.

> Not only does white sugar provide nothing really indispensable, but it also consumes some of the goodness provided by other foods.

KEY FACTS

* There are rapid-release sugars and slow-release sugars.

* Rapid-release sugars sometimes cause hypoglycaemia, which leads to headaches.

* Above all, avoid white sugar, honey, cakes and biscuits, confectionery and chocolate.

04

eat well, feel better

Our bodies need energy to function: in other words, sugar. To avoid hypoglycaemia and the headaches it causes, without depriving your body of anything it needs, eat wholegrain cereals.

Bread, pasta and rice

Slimming diets have got a lot to answer for. To reduce our calorie intake, we are encouraged to stop eating essential foods such as bread, pasta and rice – the very things that enable headache sufferers to do without white sugar safely. These foods should be consumed in as unrefined state as possible. As in the case of sugar, refining removes some essential

●●● DID YOU KNOW? —————————

> The speed at which carbohydrates pass into the bloodstream is called the glycaemic index.

> Foods with a high glycaemic index should be avoided in favour of those with a low index.

nutrients and speeds up the metabolism of sugars. Gradually substitute all the rapid-release sugars you eat with slow-release ones.

Throughout the day

- **Breakfast:** avoid all white sugar; eat wholegrain cereals instead. Avoid sweetened drinks and choose wholemeal bread or cereals.
- **Lunch:** try eating some pasta, rice or potatoes, or at least one slice of wholemeal bread.
- **Tea:** avoid all sugary foods with the exception of fruit.
- **Dinner:** eat a portion of pasta, rice, pulses or vegetables that contain sugar (such as carrots, turnips, peas).
- **Evening:** avoid eating sugary snacks in front of the television!

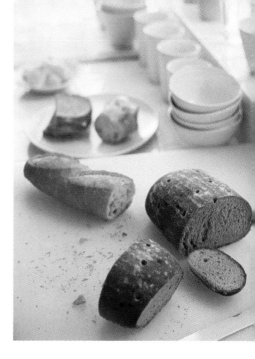

> Examples of the first group are honey, white sugar, confectionery and chocolate. In the second group are nuts (almonds, walnuts and hazelnuts), legumes (beans, lentils) and cereals (millet, oats, maize, pasta and bread). There's plenty to choose from.

KEY FACTS

* Your body needs glucose (sugar) to function.

* To provide it with all it needs while avoiding white sugar, eat cereals, dried fruits and legumes (peas, beans).

* Avoid rapid-release sugars at breakfast and eat a portion of pasta or cereals (rice, wheat) as part of your evening meal.

05

stop smoking and stay stopped

It's an obvious thing to do but not everyone does it. In addition to all the other damage it does to the body, tobacco is often a cause of headaches. So if you haven't already given up smoking, do so right away.

Smoking aggravates headaches

When you've got a bad headache, the mere smell of a cigarette is enough to turn you against the very thought of smoking. For some people this is enough, but hardened smokers light up again as soon as the headache is over. They're making a big mistake, because smoking can be a cause of headaches. Several substances in tobacco, particularly nicotine, constrict the blood vessels in the brain, which can bring on attacks.

● ● ● DID YOU KNOW?

> Beware of putting on weight when you give up smoking. Smokers tend to replace the oral satisfaction of a cigarette by constant snacking.

> To avoid this, plan other activities, such as taking up a sport, learning to paint or play a musical instrument.

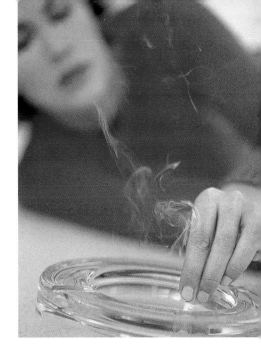

Every method has something to offer

If you've decided to stop smoking, don't hesitate to get help.

Ask your pharmacist for advice. There's a whole range of products to help you kick the habit, such as patches and nicotine chewing gum. They won't perform miracles but they may help you to stick at it during the early days.

Support groups and supervised programmes are also useful if you're worried you'll give in straight away.

Psychological support may sometimes be necessary in order to discover the hidden causes of your habit.

Finally, don't forget that natural treatments such as acupuncture, auriculotherapy, homeopathy, sophrology and even hypnotism might help.

> It's not easy to give up smoking, especially if you've had the habit for many years. It needs determination and commitment.

 KEY FACTS

* Several substances in tobacco, including nicotine, provoke headaches by narrowing the walls of blood vessels.

* Don't try to stop smoking all on your own. Seek help or advice.

* To avoid putting on weight, look for other ways of filling the gap apart from eating.

06 fatty acids are food for thought

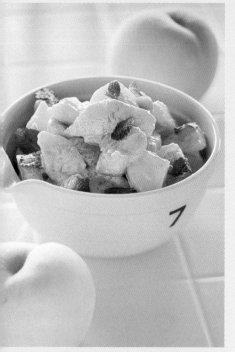

To work well, your brain needs fats. If deprived of these essential nutrients, it won't function properly. To make sure your brain is always in peak condition, learn to give it what it needs.

Brain cells love fats …

When it comes to avoiding headaches, nothing should be left to chance. Life is much less difficult if your brain is well looked after. The brain consumes a lot of essential fatty acids. These nutrients, which are contained in dietary fats, are the main constituents of nerve membranes. When the brain cells do not get enough of them, they stiffen and transmit messages less efficiently. To improve memory and concentration while reducing the stress and mental fatigue that leads to headaches, you need to consume a sufficient amount of fats, whatever the scales may say.

… but not just any fats!

Dietary fats are not all identical. Far from it. Animal fats (butter, high-fat cheeses, also fatty meats and meat products) are rich in saturated fatty acids, which raise the cholesterol level. On the other hand, fish and vegetable oils contain monounsaturated and polyunsaturated fatty acids, which feed the cell membranes without blocking the arteries.

• Reduce your intake of fatty meats (rib steaks, pork, lamb and so on).

• Instead, choose poultry, which is less fatty and, above all, fish.

• Replace butter with vegetable oils (olive, rapeseed, corn, grapeseed), which you can vary as much as you want to enjoy the different tastes and to benefit from their different constituents.

• It's best not to heat these oils as the essential fatty acids are delicate and liable to lose some of their goodness.

> These oils are rich in unsaturated fatty acids.

KEY FACTS

∗ Your brain needs certain fats in order to function well.

∗ Avoid animal fats (butter, red meat, pork, lamb) and opt for poultry, fish and uncooked vegetable oils instead.

∗ You can also take regular supplements of fish, borage and evening primrose oil in capsule form.

07

cleanse with clay

Headaches are sometimes caused by an accumulation of toxic substances. This occurs when the body is unable to get rid of waste materials as quickly and thoroughly as necessary. Clay can help with internal cleansing.

Back to earth

The body functions like any machine that uses energy: it uses fuel and it produces waste. The liver, kidneys, lungs and skin function as waste disposal organs but they are sometimes overwhelmed by the task. It doesn't help when you eat badly, get stressed or take little exercise. The result is a body clogged with waste, so that you become tired, sleep badly, feel agitated and suffer from headaches.

● ● ● DID YOU KNOW?

> If the idea of drinking clay dissolved in water disgusts you, mix powdered clay with a little water to form a quite thick paste and then roll it into some little clay balls the size of a pea.

> Leave them to dry in the sun. Take four little clay balls with a glass of water, just as you would any tablets.

For thousands of years clay has been used to purify the body. This earth is extraordinarily absorbent: it draws in harmful substances and eliminates them. Red, white or green clay – they all have therapeutic properties.

Drinking clay

Clay is most effective in liquid form. Every evening for two or three weeks, pour a dessertspoonful of clay powder into a glass of pure water (ideally, spring water with a low mineral content). Leave to soak overnight.

The following morning, drink the water from the glass without stirring it, leaving behind the clay deposit that has formed during the night. If you feel brave enough, you can stir it all in before drinking. This is more effective, but some people just can't bear the taste.

This treatment can be repeated at least once every three months, and it will rid the body of toxins and therefore eliminate your headaches, while at the same time boosting your reserves of essential minerals.

If you are on regular medication check with your doctor or pharmacist that the clay will not prevent it being absorbed from the stomach.

Warning: never use metal utensils (spoons or container).

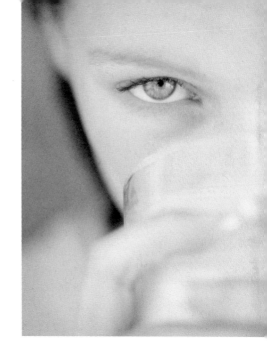

 KEY FACTS

* An accumulation of toxins in the body can sometimes cause headaches.

* To help your body cleanse itself and eliminate toxins, regularly take a course of clay in liquid form .

* If you find the taste disagreeable, make some little balls of clay and swallow them like tablets.

08 keep regular mealtimes

The body has its own rhythms of sleeping, waking, eating and so on. Certain times are better than others for each of the tasks it performs.

Night or day? The body must perform an enormous number of functions and to do so successfully it needs to be organized. For instance, there are optimum times, either at night or during the day, in the morning or the evening, for producing hormones, gastric juices and neurotransmitters. Of course, if you ask your body to produce particular substances when it is not used to doing so, it will respond but will produce smaller amounts and take longer to do it.

Keep to your usual mealtimes and your food will do you more good. Missing meals may make your blood sugar drop and make you more prone to headaches. Fatty food, alcohol and coffee, combined with eating late, make indigestion and heartburn more likely as well increasing your chances of headache.

To avoid this risk, listen to your body. Try to conform to what it tells you. And don't chop and change your mealtimes.

●●● DID YOU KNOW?

> Some people shift their daily routines. Their bodies make great efforts to adapt and then find it difficult to go back to normal. Don't push your body needlessly by requiring it to change suddenly from one rhythm to another at weekends and during the holidays.

KEY FACTS

∗ Your body has its own rhythms. If you frustrate them, it may react with headaches, etc.

∗ Try to work out which routines suit your body best.

09 no missed meals

Going without food for more than a day causes various discomforts, including headaches. Without food, the body changes the way it functions. If you don't fast, you won't run this risk.

The body slows down When forced to go without food, the body begins by using the nutrients that it finds available, mostly glycogen in the liver, which is broken down to sugar and released into the bloodstream. The body then goes into slow motion and draws from its reserves, which is strictly necessary and normally harmless, apart from the fact that in some people this may cause headaches.

Don't starve your body of food Don't make your body go without the nourishment it needs. If you are susceptible to headaches, fasting is not for you.
Eat regularly and have a snack handy if you have to skip a meal.

KEY FACTS

* When the body is no longer being nourished, blood sugar may drop.

* A drop in blood-sugar levels can cause headaches.

* To avoid this, don't skip meals or embark upon a fasting regime.

Some people suffer from headaches when they become constipated. To avoid this problem, make sure you eat the right amount of fibre.

10

fill up
with fibre

Indigestible but indispensable

When we eat plant foods and their products, most of what we eat is digested and metabolized but some of it, the fibre, is not. Fibre is, however, far from useless, since it affects the consistency and size of the stool. If there is a lack of fibre, not enough waste matter passes through the digestive system to the colon. The stool then becomes hard, dry and difficult to expel. This results in constipation and can lead to headaches in some people.

● ● ● DID YOU KNOW? ───────

> If you do eat a small amount of fibre, don't change your diet too suddenly or you're liable to upset your digestive system.

> Add fibre gradually: increase your daily intake by 10g ($^1/_2$oz) one week, then a further 10g ($^1/_2$oz) the following week. Continue in this way until you are eating a reasonable amount (about 40g/1$^1/_2$oz per day).

Moreover, fibre absorbs water and excess fats. Adding fibre to a very rich meal will prevent your intestines from becoming sluggish.

40g (1¹/₂oz) a day

Make sure you eat enough fibre and try to eat about 40g (1¹/₂oz) per day. These foods have the highest fibre content:
- **pod vegetables:** soya beans, lentils, broad beans, chickpeas, beans (17g/¹/₂oz per 100g/3¹/₂oz).
- **wholemeal cereals:** wholemeal bread, maize, millet, buckwheat, rye (10g/¹/₂oz per 100g/3¹/₂oz).
- **dried fruit:** dates, prunes, dried apricots, raisins, dried figs (10g/¹/₂oz per 100g/3¹/₂oz).
- **olives and nuts:** such as peanuts, pistachios, almonds and hazelnuts (8g/¹/₄oz per 100g/3¹/₂oz).

> It's best not to increase your intake by taking fibre in tablet form, as, unlike dietary fibre, this can disturb your digestion.

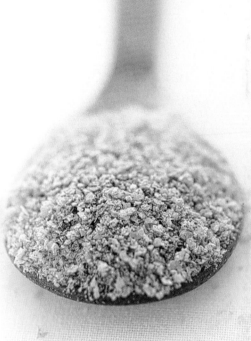

KEY FACTS

∗ Some people get headaches as soon as their intestines become sluggish.

∗ You need to eat a sufficient quantity of dietary fibre to avoid constipation.

∗ Fibre is found in wholemeal cereals, pod vegetables, dried fruit and nuts.

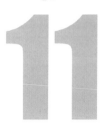

11

look after your internal bacteria

You need to look after your digestive system if it is to work well. The bacteria in your intestines will do a very good job as long as you don't ill-treat them. Find out how to pamper them, especially if you're susceptible to headaches caused by bad digestion.

Intestinal bacteria are fragile

The human gut contains billions of bacteria that help to digest food. They reproduce in the digestive tract and break down food tissue. However, like every living organism, they are fragile. Too much stress, a course of antibiotics or an unbalanced diet can seriously deplete them. Sluggish digestion, like constipation, can lead to headaches, if you happen to be susceptible.

● ● ● DID YOU KNOW?

> Whey in liquid, powder or granule form is available in health food shops.

> Whey contains essential nutrients that enable the whole body, especially the digestive system, to function properly.

Eat yoghurt

To avoid such problems, treat your bacteria as welcome guests.

• Eat one or two yoghurts daily: they contain bifidus bacteria cultures beneficial to digestion. Yoghurt is simply milk thickened to a custard-like consistency by these acid-forming bacteria. The bacteria have already begun to break down the protein molecules into lactic acid, making it easier for the body to absorb.

• Don't throw away the whey (the colourless liquid you sometimes find on the top of the yoghurt); it contains a variety of substances that are very good for the intestines.

• The fresher the yogurt, the more viable bacteria it contains, so always make sure your yoghurt is as fresh as possible. You could consider investing in a yoghurt maker, which will enable to have fresh yoghurt always on hand, at a much more reasonable cost than buying it ready-made.

• Products using probiotics, including the small dairy drinks readily available nowadays in most supermarkets, top up the system with lactic acid bacteria and support the work of beneficial bacteria already in the gut.

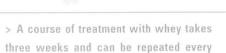

> A course of treatment with whey takes three weeks and can be repeated every three months.

KEY FACTS

∗ The intestines work well if the bacteria they contain are well looked after.

∗ Eat one or two yoghurts a day to aid the digestive system.

∗ Don't throw away the whey. The bacteria love it!

12

relax!

How about taking some of the pressure off?
Headaches are sometimes your body's way
of telling you to relax. What could be simpler?
Dim the lights, take the telephone off the
hook, stretch out and drift away ...

Autogenic training

Stress and nervous tension can trigger headaches and make them worse. To soothe them away as soon as they start, it's sometimes necessary to slow down your mind and nervous system. It was precisely to enable his patients to reach a state of muscular and mental relaxation at will that prompted Dr Schultz in the 1920s to create a technique he called 'autogenic training'. It is based on

●●● DID YOU KNOW?

> Autogenic training can also be a genuine form of psychotherapy.

> With the help of a specialized therapist, you can explore the hidden causes of very stubborn headaches.

a simple principle: a state of mental and physical relaxation can be induced and maintained by repeating a key sentence. If you practise the exercises regularly (ten minutes every morning and evening to begin with), the body and mind will eventually respond to the messages. After a few weeks you will only need to say the key sentence in your head and you'll create the desired state of mind.

Controlling pain to prevent it from developing

Lie down comfortably, eyes half-closed, in a peaceful, well-aired, dimly lit room.
• Try to achieve a state of inner calm. When you feel completely comfortable and relaxed, say silently to yourself: 'I am completely calm'.
• Feel each part of your body growing heavier: shoulders, arms, legs. Repeat in turn: 'I feel my shoulders (arms, legs, etc.) growing heavy'.
• Feel yourself growing warm, the regular beating of your heart, a cool breeze on your forehead. Repeat in turn the sentences corresponding to these sensations.

These are the basic principles. As for curing headaches, there are specific exercises that can be used as soon as you feel the first stirrings of pain, in fact as soon as you feel the very earliest warning signs. In this way you'll be able to stop the pain from developing almost before it has begun.

> The sessions also include discussions with the therapist to bring old problems and buried emotional scars out into the open.

KEY FACTS

∗ Stress and anxiety aggravate headaches.

∗ Autogenic training is a simple technique that enables you to relax at will whenever you feel the need.

13

loosen up

To avoid headaches, you need to learn to relax your body and to loosen up your muscles. There are various ways of doing this, including a technique known as eutonia, developed by Gerda Alexander in the 1950s.

The theory

The word 'eutonia' means 'harmonious tension'. The aim of this technique is to help you find just the right amount of tension for each of your bodily movements. Gerda Alexander, a German musician and director, suffered health problems from the age of 17 which limited her movements. She therefore investigated different ways of saving her

● ● ● D I D Y O U K N O W ?

> Focusing on the body in this way also allows you to relax specific areas that are over-worked as a result of poor posture.

> To cure headaches, you need to concentrate attention on the neck area, which is often the source of the pain.

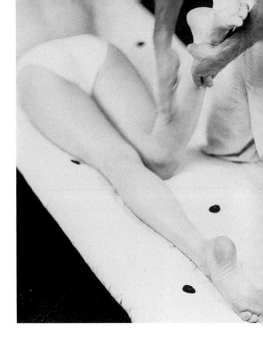

energy in order to allow her body to do as much as possible in spite of her difficulties.

Putting it into practice

During the first sessions, you will learn to be attentive to your body and to explore all its sensations. For example, you lie motionless and gradually try to become fully conscious of your arm touching the ground, of the blood flowing through your veins, of the tendons pulling upon your bones. In this way you learn to increase bodily awareness.

Little by little, in the course of the sessions, you return to the vertical position. You then focus on, for instance, tiny movements, slow-motion movements and the purpose of each of the movements. The aim is not to learn readymade solutions but to discover ones suited to the needs of each individual. A well-prepared movement, adapted to its purpose and situation, liberates and saves energy instead of using it up and wasting it.

At the same time you will also learn how to handle your physical sensations better, beginning with pain.

 KEY FACTS

* To avoid headaches, you need to learn to relax physically as well as mentally.

* There are numerous different techniques that teach muscular relaxation.

* Eutonia teaches you to be aware of your body movements so that each one is perfectly appropriate, thus liberating your energy instead of exhausting it.

14

breathe the oriental way

There's nothing better for stopping the onset of pain than to concentrate on your breathing. This relieves physical and mental tension, cleans the airways, improves the flow of oxygen in the body and, above all, makes you think about your breathing rather than the pain.

There's more than one way to breathe

Breathing is the only involuntary physical activity that can be altered at will. When we choose to, we can control our breathing and improve both our physical and psychological well being. When you breathe calmly and deeply, you feel calmer, your heart beats more regularly and slowly and your blood pressure goes down: all factors that help to get rid of a developing headache.

But you must breathe 'well'. We usually breathe in the most superficial way, so that the air penetrates the upper part of the lungs only and then is quickly expelled. However, if we use our abdominal muscles to pull down our diaphragm, we allow our chest to expand. The amount of air absorbed is much greater, the breath lasts longer and more oxygen reaches the body. What is more, breathing like this requires conscious control: when we're thinking about breathing, we think less about pain.

Breathe in, breathe out

Deep-breathing exercises almost all originate from oriental disciplines, particularly yoga.

• Sit comfortably with your back very straight and your mouth closed, and focus your attention on your nostrils.

• Breath calmly and gently through your nose, concentrating entirely on the air softly touching your nostrils as it comes and goes.

• When you breathe in, fill up your lungs so that your abdomen expands. Hold your breath for two or three seconds and then release it slowly without forcing. Concentrate on the long, slow out-breath.

• When your lungs are completely empty, wait four or five seconds before breathing in again.

After a few minutes you will notice that your breathing has become slower and more even, making your body and mind feel calmer.

KEY FACTS

∗ Learn to breathe deeply from the abdomen. This is the most simple and effective way of controlling and getting rid of a headache before it takes hold.

∗ This deep breathing technique originated in oriental disciplines such as yoga.

∗ It enables you to relax and dispel stress.

> Don't forget to breathe through the nose: the mucus membranes of the nose moisten the air in preparation for its entry into the lungs and the cilia (little hairs) that line the nose rid the air of impurities.

Increased blood pressure can cause headaches. Even if you don't suffer from chronically high blood pressure, keep a regular eye on it. Stress, worries and problems can cause a temporary increase, which could result in headaches.

15

watch your blood pressure

The rhythm of your heartbeat

Blood pressure readings measure the pressure exerted by the blood on the artery walls as it is pumped around the body by the heart. They consist of two figures. The first, the higher figure, represents the pressure when the heart contracts (the systolic pressure) to propel the blood. The second figure represents the pressure when the heart relaxes

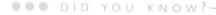

● ● ● DID YOU KNOW?

> Only chronic cases of raised blood pressure need to be treated with drugs.

> When blood pressure is permanently too high, medication is the only way to keep it under control.

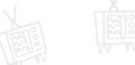

(the diastolic pressure). Normal pressures should be less than 140/90 and even lower in younger people.

Damage can be caused if blood pressure rises above these figures: the artery walls become less and less elastic and can sometimes end by breaking, with serious consequences. The long-term risks are strokes, heart disease and damage to the kidneys.

High blood pressure (hypertension) itself often has no obvious symptoms and is detected only at a check up, but it may be associated with head pain, and rapid rises in blood pressure to high levels can cause severe headaches.

Keeping your blood pressure down

Even if you're not normally hypertensive, your blood pressure can temporarily rise in moments of stress. If you tend to get headaches when you are tired and tense, check whether or not the attacks are due to high blood pressure. If they are, learn to relax. Try yoga, relaxation or breathing techniques. Or you could try a more in-depth treatment, such as homeopathy, herbal medicine or acupuncture.

> However, this kind of treatment may have side effects, which is why prevention is better than cure. It is preferable to try less drastic measures first.

KEY FACTS

* Headaches are sometimes triggered by a rise in blood pressure.

* Temporary increases can sometimes result from stress and tiredness.

* Chronically high blood pressure should be treated by a doctor in order to prevent complications.

16 keep an even temperature

Some weather conditions cause headaches, especially sudden changes in temperature. So, if you're susceptible to headaches, avoid them.

Narrowing and widening of the blood vessels The body employs a very sophisticated system known as homeostasis, which is designed to maintain body temperature at a stable level. When it experiences a sudden change of temperature, the body adjusts to it by temporarily widening or narrowing blood vessels and altering blood flow in the skin and scalp to lose or conserve heat. Sometimes these sudden changes in blood flow can be associated with headaches while the body adapts to the new level. Changes to the size of blood vessels in the brain can cause temporary headaches.

Avoid saunas, steam rooms and very hot baths If you're liable to this type of reaction, avoid sudden exposure to very low or very high temperatures. Always try to pass gradually from one extreme to the other. Don't undress all at once when you enter a very hot room.

●●● DID YOU KNOW?

> Some people can suffer violent but very brief headaches (lasting a few seconds) when they eat ice cream. This is probably due to the sudden cold temperatures in the mouth stimulating the nerves in the teeth and gums.

KEY FACTS

* The body needs time to adapt to sudden changes in temperature.

* Headaches can be triggered when blood vessels widen or narrow.

17 choose your wine carefully

For reasons of taste you should never drink poor-quality wine and there's all the more reason to avoid it if you suffer from headaches. Bad wine can cause headaches: the poorer the quality, the more rapid and intense the headaches.

Red or white wine? The French think it's white wine that causes headaches, whilst in Britain it's red wine that gets the blame. Why the difference? It's not very clear. What we do know, however, is that alcoholic drinks contain substances such as histamine, tyramine and phenols, which cause the blood vessels to swell. Some migraine sufferers find that wine is a trigger for their headaches.

Tannins and chemical products One thing is certain, however, that good-quality wines cause fewer headaches. This is partly due to the absence of certain chemicals that are added to cheaper wines. It is also true that light red wines cause headaches less often than heavy, heady ones and the fact remains that some sufferers tolerate white wine less well than red.

● ● ● DID YOU KNOW?

> You should never drink more than the recommended limits (three glasses a day for men, two glasses for women, with one or two drink-free days a week). More than this, and the benefits of the wine (protection against heart disease) are outweighed by the damage done by the alcohol. Wine should always be consumed in moderation.

KEY FACTS

∗ Wine can give some people headaches, although it's not clear precisely why.

∗ Poor-quality wines are much more likely to be guilty of this than good-quality ones.

18

Chinese medicine attributes headaches to an imbalance in the flow of energy. To remedy this, the Chinese regularly practise Qi Gong, a very ancient form of gymnastics that regulates the circulation of energy in the body.

s-t-r-e-t-c-h

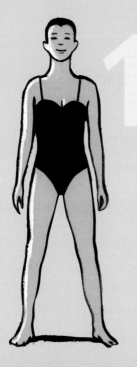

1

Too much or too little

According to Chinese medicine, good health depends on the even circulation of vital energy throughout the body. This energy, which feeds all our organs, flows through currents called meridians. If there is too little or too much energy, imbalances occur that cause problems like headaches.

Headaches often occur when there is too much or too little vital energy in the heart meridian. However, there is an exercise to adjust the flow of energy in the heart.

Stretching the heart meridian

① Stand with legs slightly bent, feet a little apart and back straight.

② Cross your arms in front of your chest, making sure your forearms, wrists and fingers are quite relaxed.

③ Keeping your arms outstretched, raise them to surround your head, palms facing upwards.

④ Stretch the little finger and the outer edge of each hand before lowering your arms to your sides.

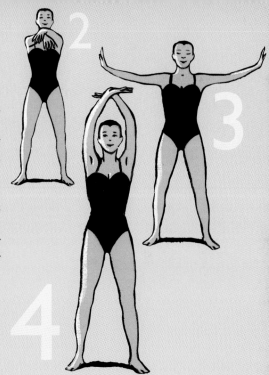

● ● ● DID YOU KNOW?

> You must be in a state of mental relaxation when performing Qi Gong exercises: breathe calmly for a few minutes before beginning and continue to concentrate on your breathing throughout the exercise. Try to empty your mind of other thoughts and visualize the energy passing through your body and nourishing your organs.

KEY FACTS

* In Chinese medicine headaches are often attributed to an imbalance of energy in the heart meridian.

* Performing a Qi Gong exercise helps to regulate this energy.

* Relax before the exercise, breathe calmly and concentrate on what is happening in your body.

19

move that body!

Sport is a good way of getting rid of stress, tension and toxins. In other words, besides helping you to feel good and stay healthy, it's also a way of avoiding headaches.

Less tension, fewer headaches

The benefits of sport are now well known. A regular and reasonable amount of physical activity reduces anxiety, helps you to sleep, keeps the cardiovascular system in good shape, enables more oxygen to reach the tissues, increases lung power, promotes the circulation of lymph fluids and the removal of waste matter, improves digestion, loosens the joints and so on and so on. Besides all

● ● ● DID YOU KNOW?

> You can always find ways of exercising on a daily basis.

> Merely walking to the shops, provided they're at least 30 minutes away, or climbing the stairs instead of taking the lift are useful forms of exercise, especially if that's all you normally get.

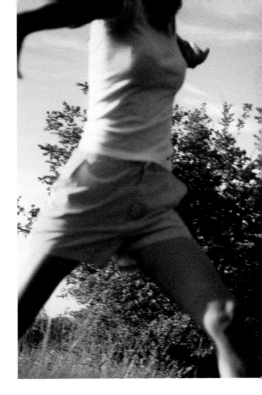

this, it can cure certain kinds of head-ache as well, particularly those due to stress, an accumulation of toxins or circulation problems.

Doing yourself good doesn't have to be painful

Sport need not mean competition. The most important thing is to enjoy it. There's nothing to be gained from forc-ing yourself to go at a crazy pace. Blood, sweat and tears do not mean that you're doing yourself good.

It's best to choose a sport that works the whole body gently, such as walking, slow jogging, swimming or cycling. Regularity is what really matters: forty minutes two or three times a week is a good average. However, a regular session just once a week is better than trying it for a little while and then giving up.

> If you haven't done any sport for a long time and have any doubts about your fitness, check with a doctor before you undertake any activity. Some sports have specific contraindications: a weak heart, back and joint problems.

KEY FACTS

* Among its many benefits, exercise gets rid of stress, improves blood circulation and speeds up the elimination of waste from the body.

* Choose a sport or exercise you enjoy, use your car less and always take the stairs.

20 negative ions are a positive thing

We all have to breathe but, ideally, it should be healthy, pure, unpolluted air, air that is, above all, rich in negative ions, which are as good for us as vitamins. To do this, there's nothing better than walks in the country.

Positive ions and negative ions When we breathe, we draw in various gases, particularly oxygen. Oxygen atoms are charged with electricity, some positive, some negative. Negative ions do us good and if we don't absorb enough of them, we may be liable to suffer from tiredness, insomnia and headaches.

Get out in the country The problem is that negative ions are much more fragile than positive ones and they are rapidly destroyed when indoors. There are several ways that you can get round this problem:
• Air your house regularly. Keeping your windows open for just five minutes is enough to clean up the air in an average-sized room.
• Go for country walks.
• Buy an ionizer: these little devices produce negative ions.

KEY FACTS
* We need to breathe in negative ions to be healthy.

* To get enough of them, air your home and take walks in the country.

* Buying an ionizer is another option.

case study

As the manager of a finance department, Carol can't afford to make the slightest mistake at work and she certainly can't allow herself to be absent frequently. Consequently, she has learnt to 'manage' her headaches. 'As soon as I suspected that I could be a regular headache sufferer,' she said, 'I consulted a specialist. I drew up a battle plan with him, because I've no wish to suffer from headaches and, in any case, I haven't the time. First of all, we worked out a special diet. Then I did something about getting enough physical activity. I hate sport but I'm very happy to go for long walks on the beach. Finally, I learnt a relaxation technique that enables me to relax for a few minutes wherever I am, whenever I feel tension or a migraine coming on. This short break allows my body to take charge and solve the problem. I don't really know how it does it but the upshot is that the migraine I thought I was going to get doesn't materialize.'

21 »»

»» **Changing your lifestyle to avoid headaches** may be helpful, but if they continue there's no point in simply suffering in silence.

»»» **If, despite your best intentions and new habits,** you still get headaches, stop them from hurting as soon as they show signs of starting. There's no need to resort to conventional painkillers with their side effects. Take them only in an emergency.

»»»» **Plants, massage and eye yoga** are among the natural ways of taking away the pain.

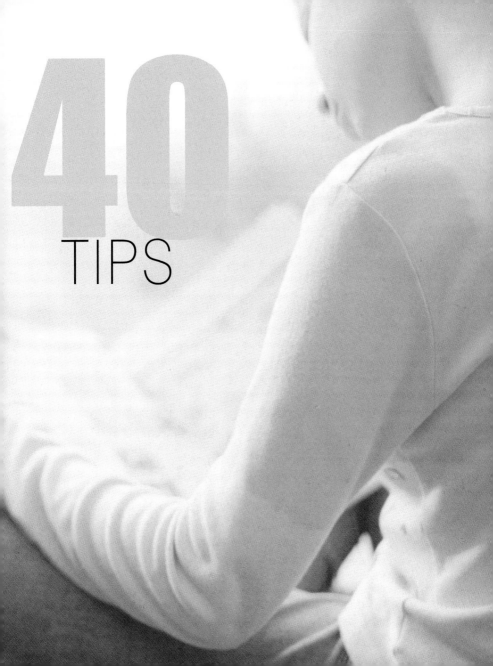

40
TIPS

21

calm is what you need

Can't get rid of your headaches? There's one thing you must do: make sure those you live with understand what you're going through and give you some peace and quiet.

Avoid noise and bright light

When you feel a headache coming on there's nothing more upsetting than noise, whether it's traffic in the street or the loud music your son is listening to in his bedroom. Loud noise always makes a headache worse and so does bright light. General commotion, comings and goings, doors slamming and so on, are just as bad for you. Put a stop to it now!

● ● ● DID YOU KNOW?

> When a headache comes during the working day, it may be impossible to rest completely but you can adopt a defence strategy: isolate yourself as much as possible from others after explaining why and try to work as calmly as possible at your own pace.

> Move about as little as possible. Avoid disagreements with your colleagues: if necessary, give in to them even when they're wrong – you can put them right tomorrow!

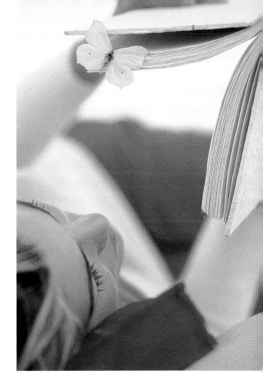

Ask others to quieten down and show some consideration for your pain. If you can rest immediately, away from noise, light and movement, you'll have a better chance of putting an end to that piercing sensation in your head.

Curtains, masks, ear plugs

• Choose the quietest room in the house. If you get frequent headaches, it's worth insulating the room against noise (double glazing, fabric draping the walls), so you can take refuge there as soon as you feel the need.
• Make it as dark as possible: close the shutters and curtains.
• If necessary, use earplugs to block out surrounding noises and a black mask to protect your eyes from the light.
• Lie down, make yourself as comfortable as possible and rest.
• Above all, don't feel guilty about imposing strict rules on your household. You have to. It's to everyone's advantage that your headache goes away: your nearest and dearest will then find you serene and happy again instead of suffering and grumpy!

 KEY FACTS

∗ Settle down in a quiet room away from noise, disturbance and light.

∗ Ask your household to show you some consideration.

∗ If necessary, use earplugs and an eye-mask that won't let the light through.

22
camomile can help

Camomile has been used for centuries to treat headaches. There are several varieties, all of which have similar effects. However, the most effective as a cure for headaches is German camomile, also known as mayweed.

Long, long ago

German camomile (*Matricaria* or 'true' *recutita*) was widely used in Ancient Greece, when it was discovered to have several medicinal properties that have been scientifically confirmed nineteen hundred years later. It was mainly used then as a means of regulating menstrual flow and easing period headaches. Its use as a cure for headache pains gradually spread to other countries.

● ● ● DID YOU KNOW? ─────────

> Don't pick German camomile yourself. Always buy it from pharmacies or health food shops.

> If you buy the plant loose, make sure it's organic or picked in the wild.

This common plant, which is found throughout Europe along roadsides and on waste ground, is used in various forms including an infusion, a pure essential oil or a massage oil.

Using German camomile

German camomile is usually prescribed as a treatment for headaches caused by the onset of a period, fever, anxiety, facial neuralgia or digestive problems. It also aids digestion and is a light sedative.

• **Herbal tea:** add 1 spoonful of dried camomile leaves to 250ml (8fl oz) of boiling water; leave to infuse for 10 minutes. Drink a cupful in the evening before going to bed, if possible quite a long time after the last meal.

• **Pure essential oil:** put three drops (no more!) on the pads of your fingers and massage into the temples with light circular movements. You can also massage an aching forehead.

• **Massage oil:** mix German camomile essential oil with a carrier oil (grapeseed, sweet almond, jojoba) in the proportions of 5% essential oil and 95% base oil. Use a tablespoonful of the mixture to massage the whole of the face, avoiding the area around the eyes.

> Adopt the same approach when buying essential oil: choose 100% pure and natural organic products. Warning: don't exceed the recommended dose, especially if you're using the essential oil. It's very concentrated and strong.

KEY FACTS

* German camomile, or mayweed, has been used since ancient times as a treatment for headaches.

* You can use it to make a herbal tea or massage it as an essential oil into painful areas.

* Make sure you always try to buy plants that have been picked in the wild.

23 try an old wives' tale

To control the pain as soon as it starts, you might try to use some good old-fashioned remedies. They can be very effective.

Cold dulls pain Our grandmothers knew some tricks that are worth remembering. As soon as you feel the first stirrings of pain, take a cloth and a container filled with very cold water and lie down quietly in a darkened room. Wet the cloth, wring it out and put it on your forehead or the back of your neck. It should cover the whole surface from ear to ear. As soon as the cloth starts to get warm, put it back in the water and repeat the procedure.

Follow your instinct When you get a headache, you tend to rub the place where it hurts. This instinct has a sound physiological basis. Firstly, the very act of massaging a particular area stimulates the secretion of endorphins, painkilling substances that are produced by the brain. What's more, the places most frequently rubbed also correspond precisely to acupuncture points: the bridge of the nose, the temples and the base of the skull.

● ● ● DID YOU KNOW?

> If you can't bear the pain any longer, try a good old ice pack. Fill the pack with ice-cubes and place it on the painful area (back of the neck, forehead). Keep it there until the pain dies down but not for more than 10 minutes or you could cause an ice burn on your skin.

KEY FACTS

* The mere act of massaging a particular part of the body stimulates the secretion of painkilling endorphins.

* Cold compresses are a good treatment for headaches.

24 picture your pain

When you're in pain, it's worth trying any method that might relieve it, even the most eccentric. Do you know that sometimes all you need to get rid of the pain is a simple ritual? You can invent your own.

The placebo effect We have greater mental powers than we think, including a capacity for self-healing that can overcome a good many pains. A placebo is a substance that has the appearance of a drug but has no medicinal value. There really is such a thing as a placebo effect and current research is gradually coming to understand its secrets. If you firmly believe that you'll get better, you can help it to happen.

Drawing might be the answer But how to activate the placebo effect when it's needed? There's no infallible method. What follows is merely one possible answer:
• Think of your pain as something with a shape and colour that can be drawn.
• Draw it on a piece of paper.
• Then burn the drawing and ask the smoke to take the pain away with it.

KEY FACTS

* We all possess a remarkable capacity for self-healing.

* Little personal rituals can trigger this off.

* For example, make a picture of your pain and then burn it!

25

take your feet in hand

What if the solution to these headaches that are making your life a misery is right underfoot? This is what reflexologists believe: they have some surprising, simple and often effective solutions to offer.

Your whole body is influenced by your feet

Reflexology draws its inspiration from traditional Chinese medicine and its conception of the energy flow in the body. Good health is the result of the even, unblocked circulation of vital energy, whilst illnesses occur when the circulation is unbalanced.

Traditional Chinese medicine holds that the soles of our feet show a 'reflex chart' of the whole body. Each organ, energy meridian (current) and vital function corresponds to an area on the sole of the foot. By massaging particular points on this reflex chart, we can regulate the flow of energy round the body when it has been disturbed.

Massaging your feet

• To relieve sinus pains, vigorously massage the underside of your five toes, using tiny circular movements.

• Treat pains in the skull by concentrating on the underside of the two big toes, particularly the one on the left foot.

• To relieve more widespread pain, massage the whole foot: begin with the sole, working from toes to heel. Then repeat on the upper part. Do the same on the other foot. You should press energetically but lightly.

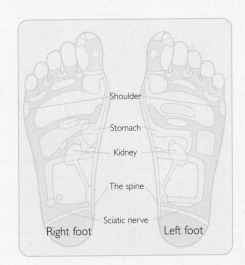

Shoulder

Stomach

Kidney

The spine

Sciatic nerve

Right foot   Left foot

KEY FACTS

∗ Reflexology is a therapy inspired by traditional Chinese medicine, which regulates energy flow.

∗ On the soles of our feet we all have a 'reflex chart' that corresponds with the various organs of the body.

∗ By massaging certain points on the feet it is possible to restore correct energy flow and relieve headaches.

26 don't dwell on the pain

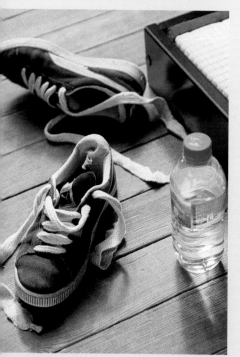

If you suffer frequently from pain, it's usually very hard to forget all about it. Even when pain-free, you can remain anxious, in case it might return. Try to get rid of this pointless and exhausting anxiety.

> You'll be living at a fast and enjoyable rate but be careful not to push things too far. If you suffer an attack, slow down, take the time to deal with it, accept its existence.

● ● ● DID YOU KNOW?

> Devise a programme of short-, medium- and long-term plans to make this technique of getting your mind to forget about pain even more effective.

Silence can be deafening

Sometimes silence can be as disturbing as a sudden outbreak of loud noise. A long-term sufferer develops a similarly paradoxical state of mind: the pain can sometimes be felt as a constant lurking threat, even when it's not there. It's far better not to think about it but sometimes that's much easier said than done. However, with a little imagination you can find enough distractions to enable you to forget it … at least until the next attack.

Get out and about

The best way of forgetting the pain is to keep busy. Physical activity will enable you to immerse yourself in the effort and forget your fears. A passion for antiques, archaeology or entomology will offer your mind new areas for exploration and discovery. Improve your social life, go out and meet new people, join a local club. This could snowball and lead you to new absorbing activities. Visits to the cinema or leisure activities with a group of friends might also form part of a program to help you get rid of the fear that 'it' will soon start up again.

> If you don't, you'll just be exchanging one problem for another.

KEY FACTS

* When the pain goes away, a long-term sufferer sometimes becomes obsessed by the fear that it will return.

* The best way of avoiding this is to keep your mind busy.

* Trips to the cinema, painting, outings with friends – in fact all enjoyable activities – will relieve this anxiety.

The mind can be fooled. When a desirable situation is convincingly imagined, we can end up believing it's really true. Some mind/body techniques make use of this fact to relieve headaches.

27

visualize a
pain-free life

Once upon a time ...

That still, small inner voice is never quiet; it is always creating scenarios, often negative or dramatic, that we end up believing in. However, many motivational and relaxation techniques use this habit to create positive images and to help resolve problems, even relieve pain. Sending positive messages to the mind when you are in a state close to sleep enables it to absorb new propositions that can modify the way in which we look at things.

Sophrology, hypnosis, visualization ...

Sophrology, hypnosis, self-hypnosis and visualization are all techniques based upon the same principle: if the resting mind is fed with positive messages, psychological or physical changes can be achieved. Each technique can reduce pain in its own way and each should be practised in a state of deep relaxation. Visualization employs mental images, hypnosis words spoken by the therapist, self-hypnosis words you speak yourself and sophrology a mixture of both words and images.

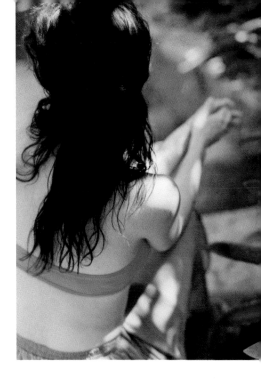

> For good measure, you can attempt to go a bit further by adding, 'I'm feeling really fit' or 'I have a memory like an elephant'. You never know!

 KEY FACTS

* Techniques such as hypnosis, visualization and sophrology enable us to receive positive messages that can relieve some forms of pain.

* It is important to always have affirmative thoughts and to create positive images in your mind.

28

release blocked energy

Chinese medicine has given rise to various therapies, all based on the same premise: since illness is the result of an imbalance in the energy flow, it can be cured when smooth circulation has been restored. Jin Shin Do, or *do-in*, enables you to do this yourself by working on particular massage points.

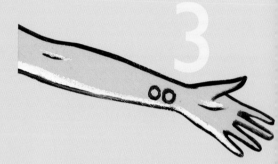

Releasing the blockage

Jin Shin Do, or *do-in*, is based on the same principles as acupuncture: you work on the energy flow by stimulating points on the meridians (energy currents) in order to restore harmonious circulation throughout the body. An acupuncturist uses needles, whereas a practitioner of Jin Shin Do uses the fingers – acupressure. You can also perform this technique upon yourself. Barehanded, first massage a large area and then concentrate on the appropriate points with your thumb or fingertips.

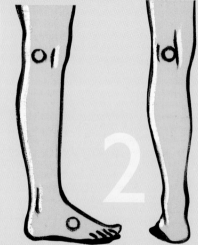

Curing a headache

As soon as the pain starts, sit down and make yourself comfortable in a quiet place, breathe deeply, close your eyes and lightly massage all your head for a minute. Next, concentrate on these points:

① If the pain is in the temples, press on the outside of the leg, level with the knee, and also a couple of inches above the fourth toe.

② If the pain is at the top of your head, massage the centre of the hollow at the back of the knee.

③ If the pain is in the forehead, concentrate on the inside of your wrist, first about an inch and then about two inches above the point where it joins the hand.

④ If the problem is at the back of your neck, press on the base of the skull and the hollow of the collarbone.

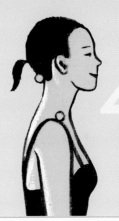

● ● ● DID YOU KNOW?

> Stimulating the points used in Jin Shin Do tones up the skin, activates the circulation of blood and lymph fluids, helps in the elimination of toxins, relieves mental and emotional tension and increases the secretion of hormones. Trust in your own sensations when looking for a particular point: the blocked point is usually painful to the touch. Stimulate it more and more vigorously as the pain dies away.

KEY FACTS

* Jin Shin Do is based on the same principles as acupuncture.

* It involves massaging with the fingers particular points situated on the energy meridians (currents).

* You can massage yourself, choosing the points to be worked on according to where you feel the pain.

29

Chinese medicine has influenced the culture of neighbouring countries. One of the techniques it has inspired is the Vietnamese therapy of Dien Cham or facial reflexology, which very rapidly relieves headaches.

try facial massage

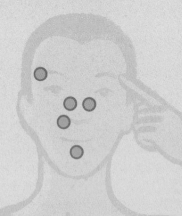

Stimulating the face

Dien Cham is not as well known as acupuncture. It is a form of reflexology involving the stimulation of particular points on the face. The more precise the points chosen, the more effective is the treatment of various medical problems, including headaches. Acupuncturists, who perform this technique, use needles whilst non-specialists use a round-tipped object, such as a pen top or the bent joint of the index finger.

All you need to do is tap the chosen place for about twenty seconds, gently at first and then more and more strongly. The more vigorous the stimulation, the more rapid the results.

Some precise Die Cham points for headaches

Here are some of the points advocated by Dien Cham therapists for curing headaches:
• To the right of the nose, just in front of the right nostril, just above where a man's moustache might be.
• Just below the lower lip in the hollow between the lip and the chin.

• On either side of the nose at the point where the nostrils begin to flare out, at the junction of the cartilage and the bone. This is the zone upon which you apply pressure when suffering from a sinusitis headache.
• At the outer end of each eyebrow: these are the places you instinctively press when a pain seems to grip you like a vice (or that you tap when you want to indicate someone is 'nuts').

● ● ● DID YOU KNOW?

> Dien Cham is based upon the principles of reflexology, in other words, the idea that certain parts of the body encapsulate, in a sense, the whole organism. Each organ has its corresponding point on the skin of the foot, the hands, the face or the ear. Stimulation of these exact points is communicated to the organ concerned, by a kind of echo. Dien Cham is not yet very widespread and there aren't many properly trained therapists. However, if you trust in your instincts and your sensations, you'll find the right points on your face perfectly well.

KEY FACTS

* Dien Cham is a Vietnamese technique of facial reflexology, which can relieve the pain associated with headaches very quickly.

* Dien Cham involves the stimulation of precise points on the face with the rounded end of a pen or with the bent joint of the index finger.

* If you are able to trust your instinct, you can easily locate the right facial points yourself.

Headaches may mean that your body is overloaded by too much alcohol and a poor diet. It's easy to find relief through the healing powers of medicinal plants.

30

look after your liver

Overload your body and your head will suffer

Headaches sometimes occur because the liver is working overtime trying to deal with a diet that is too heavy, too fatty, too sugary or too alcoholic. Not enough bile is secreted, digestion slows down, toxins accumulate and your head suffers. However plants offer a very effective means of helping the liver do its work. Some are taken in the form of herbal teas, others as capsules and still

● ● ● DID YOU KNOW?

> Black radish and dandelion are also beneficial to those suffering from a sluggish liver.

> Black radish helps drain away the waste materials that accumulate in the liver, whilst dandelion stimulates the production of bile and helps remove toxins.

others can be eaten as a salad. All of them have proved their worth over thousands of years.

The art of using herbal remedies

• **Artichoke:** benefits the liver by stimulating the production and elimination of bile and helping to renew its cells. To make a herbal infusion, pour 1 generous spoonful of dried leaves (don't use the flower) into a cup of boiling water. Drink 2 cups a day, sweetened with honey as it is very bitter. You can also eat artichokes raw or cooked.

• **Boldo:** gives the liver a tonic by stimulating the secretion of bile and activating the digestive system. To make a herbal tea, use 10g (1/2oz) of boldo per litre (1¾pints) of boiling water and drink a cup before every meal.

• **Lime sapwood** (the inner layer of bark and the wood immediately underneath it): helps a sluggish liver due to its high flavonoid content. It also relieves the headaches and nausea that arise when the liver is not functioning properly. To make a decoction, use 1 tablespoon of lime sapwood per cup of cold water and boil for 3 minutes. Drink 4 cups a day, sweetened with honey.

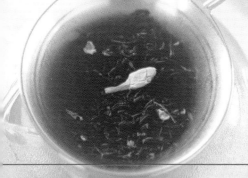

> **So don't think twice! When they're in season, eat them raw, flavoured with a good vegetable oil and a little cider vinegar or lemon juice. They do you good, they're tasty and your digestive system will thank you for them.**

KEY FACTS

∗ Headaches are often a sign that your liver is overloaded and needs to be cleansed.

∗ Artichoke, boldo, lime sapwood, black radish and dandelion are all very effective treatments. They can be made into herbal tea and/or eaten as a salad.

31

soothe
your eyes

The eyes are particularly sensitive if you suffer from headaches. Firstly, tired eyes can cause headaches and secondly, headaches are made worse by light. Whichever is your problem, you need to do something about it quickly.

Take care of your eyes

Certain kinds of bright light that would never bother most people can be painful for headache sufferers: the sun's rays through a window, a very harsh light, the setting sun over an expanse of water, the dazzle caused by car headlights at night. Sometimes even daylight can be just too strong for them. Those who spend all day looking at a computer screen are also liable to suffer from tired eyes, thus increasing the likelihood of headaches. The traditional Indian therapy of eye yoga can, however, cure these problems.

Exercises for the eyes

'Palming' is a good way of resting your eyes.

• Place your left hand over your left eye, covering the eye socket with the palm of your hand and resting your four fingers over the bridge of your nose. Put your right hand over your right eye in the same way with the fingers covering those of the other hand.

• Now no light can reach your eyes. Stay like this for several minutes, breathing deeply and relaxing your eyelids and eye muscles.

Eye yoga also has a number of specific exercises for relaxing the eyes when headaches are caused by focusing on objects that are too close. For example, stare for a few minutes at a candle flame or the end of your nose, then roll your eyeballs clockwise several times, then followed by an anti-clockwise roll several times.

To help to widen the blood vessels in your eyes and provide them with more oxygen, vigorously flutter your eyelids over and over again until tears start to run. You can repeat this exercise several times a day.

● ● ● DID YOU KNOW?

> These eye exercises are a really good way of combating stress, because relaxing the eye muscles also helps to relax other muscles in the body.

> You can also relieve eye tension and fatigue by rinsing your eyes in some soothing cornflower water. This is an ancient remedy but still remains as effective as ever.

KEY FACTS

* Eye fatigue can make headaches worse and, conversely, headaches can make eye fatigue worse.

* To break this vicious circle, try doing some eye yoga.

* These simple exercises are relaxing and improve your vision.

32 change your glasses

Headaches are sometimes due to the fact that one little detail has been overlooked for far too long – either you need glasses or the ones you have are no longer strong enough.

If you get frequent headaches that are slow to go away, you need to ask yourself the following questions. Am I suffering from tired eyes? Do I need to wear glasses or change the ones I've got? As your vision deteriorates, your eyes at first adapt to the deficiency. They struggle on with their normal functions, and the strain is not noticed immediately. It is these extra efforts that cause headaches.

As people head towards middle age, the lens becomes stiffer and can no longer change its shape to cope with near vision. Even people with previously perfect eyesight may need glasses for reading.

Have your eyesight checked regularly
Get your eyes tested even if you don't wear glasses. If you already wear them, you should consult an optometrist (optician) about once a year. They will check if your glasses are still suitable and will, if necessary, prescribe you a new pair. They can also detect other, related problems (sensitivity to light, ocular hypertension) that might make your headaches worse.

● ● ● D I D   Y O U   K N O W ?

> Eye yoga can also help (see p. 69). Specially adapted exercises will help you improve the strength and flexibility of the muscles used for focusing, thus enabling you to regain several degrees of vision.

KEY FACTS

* Headaches can be caused if your eyes are focusing less sharply.

* Consult an optometrist, who will prescribe glasses if you need them.

33 get into hot water

Here's another old trick that works well – as soon you feel the first twinges of pain, plunge your hands and feet into hot water. It's simple and effective, if you do it quickly enough.

A simple solution Do you feel the first signs of a bad headache coming on? Wherever you are, hurry to the bathroom or toilet. Fill the washbasin with hot water and immerse your hands. Leave them underwater for a few minutes while gently massaging your wrists, starting at the inside and working outwards. If possible, do the same for your feet, and massage your calves, starting from the ankles and moving slowly upwards.

A more sophisticated method A slightly more strenuous technique involves dipping your feet first into a bath of hot water for a few minutes and then, briefly into a bath of cold water. This trick has been handed down from mother to daughter for many generations and is a good way of relieving headaches caused by the menstrual cycle.

● ● ● DID YOU KNOW?

> Both methods (hot water on its own, or hot water followed by cold) improve blood circulation. The effect is rapid but not necessarily long-lasting. Fortunately, either method can be repeated safely as often as you like.

KEY FACTS

* As soon as you feel the onset of pain, plunge your hands and feet into hot water.

* Another method consists of dipping your feet first in hot water, then in cold water.

* Hot water, or hot water followed by cold water, improves blood circulation.

34

mud, glorious mud!

Natural dried clay is often used as a face mask, compress or poultice for drawing and absorbing impurities from the skin. An old remedy that has proved itself time and again, clay poultices can also help ease pain. It never fails, particularly if you add a few drops of a suitable essential oil.

Green clay and a little water

To prepare a poultice, mix some green clay with a little water, stir and add enough virgin olive oil to make a smooth paste. Spread it on a clean cloth and apply the poultice directly to your forehead or the back of your neck at the first signs of pain or during an attack. Some advise a cold poultice, others prefer it hot. If in doubt, start with a hot one and let it cool down. This way you can establish which method works best for you.

Add a few drops of essential oil

You could add a few drops of essential oils to the clay paste before spreading it on the cloth to make it even more soothing. Here is a mixture that works well:
• 5 drops of lavender essential oil (*Lavandula officinalis*)
• 5 drops of sage (*Salvia officinalis*)
• 5 drops of oregano (*Origanum vulgare*)
Blend well and then proceed as before. The essential oils will diffuse slowly into the cloth and the skin, helping to relieve the pain.
Clay can also be stirred into water and drunk to help cleanse the digestive tract (see p. 25).

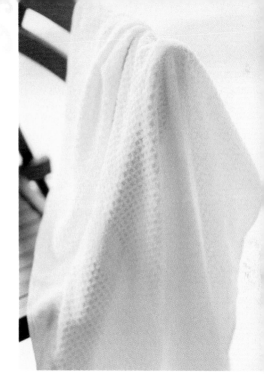

> Above all, don't use metal, because it affects the clay and reduces its effectiveness.

KEY FACTS

* You can prepare clay poultices to relieve your headaches.

* Add a few drops of essential oil to the clay poultice: lavender, sage, oregano.

* The poultices can be used hot or cold: choose the temperature that suits you best.

35

boost your digestive system

Good internal hygiene is vital if you want to stay healthy. If you frequently get headaches, it could be due to an overloaded digestive system. A slight adjustment of your diet and a few plants can help.

The natural way

If a sluggish digestive system is causing your headaches, avoid chemical laxatives at all costs. Millions of laxatives are sold every year. They may solve the problem in the short term but in the long run they make it worse, because they are irritants. What's more, some of them cause artificial contractions of the colon and can cause colicky pain. Long-term

> The walls of the intestines need to be strong and flexible if they are to do their work properly. To help achieve this, take regular exercise but don't overdo it. Choose activities like walking, swimming or cycling.

> These activities have a massaging effect on the abdominal region and improve bowel movements. Some yoga exercises are also very helpful.

use can damage the colon. It's better, firstly, to consider whether your diet is to blame (see p. 14) and, if so, to try a herbal cure. These plants are not laxatives in the true sense of the word but they will tone up your intestines without irritating them.

Plants that benefit the intestines

Plants that revive intestinal activity: mallow (*Malva sylvestris*), marsh mallow (*Althea officinalis*) and alder buckthorn (*Rhamnus frangula*).

• Mallow is not actually a laxative but has soothing and calming properties. Infuse a tablespoonful of leaves and flowers for 10 minutes in 250ml (8fl oz) of hot water. Drink up to 3 cupfuls a day.

• Marsh mallow has a similar calming effect on irritated, inflamed intestines. Use 15g (1/2oz) of leaves per 250ml (8fl oz) of boiling water and infuse for 10 minutes. Drink up to 3 cupfuls a day.

• Alder buckthorn has greater laxative qualities and can be used when you're really constipated. Use a teaspoonful of the plant per 250ml (8fl oz) of cold water, boil for 5 minutes and infuse for 10 minutes. Drink a cupful in the evening at bedtime.

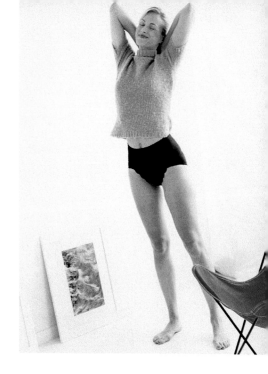

KEY FACTS

∗ Some plants are very effective in treating sluggish intestines, a condition often responsible for recurrent headaches.

∗ Mallow, marsh mallow and alder buckthorn relieve intestinal problems.

∗ Avoid laxatives and take regular exercise.

36

You're ready to party with friends. You've thought about what you're going to eat, what you're going to wear and ... how you're going to look after your body! Here's how to avoid a splitting headache the morning after.

no more morning-after

Herbal teas and homeopathy

You're going to be eating and drinking a lot, dancing, exposed to a variety of strong smells and possibly spending several hours in a smoky atmosphere. To avoid waking up feeling sick and with a headache, prepare for what, of course, will be a very enjoyable occasion, but one that can sometimes have undesirable consequences. Here are some precautions to take before leaving home.

● ● ● DID YOU KNOW?

> Some therapists advise drinking a tablespoonful of olive oil an hour or two before the meal.

> This gives the stomach walls a fatty lining that enables heavy foods to pass through more easily.

> You could also drink clay 'milk' for three or four days after the party (see p.25).

• Prepare a soothing herbal tea for when you get back (just in case!): 20g (³/₄oz) of meadowsweet (*Spiraea ulmaria*), 60g (2¹/₂oz) of blackcurrant (*Ribes nigrum*) and 30g (1oz) of ash (*Fraxinus excelsior*), infused in 1 litre (1³/₄pints) of hot water. Drink one cupful, or more if necessary.

• As for a homeopathic remedy, a few hours before your party take a dose of *Nux Vomica* 7C.

During the party

• Go prepared. Keep a little bottle containing 10ml (¹/₂fl oz) of peppermint (*Mentha piperita*) essential oil in your pocket. If you feel a headache coming on, rub one or two drops onto your temples and the back of your neck: this will ensure a pleasant feeling of freshness and pain relief.

• During the meal, avoid too many mixtures and keep to one kind of drink, ideally the best red wine available or a very dry white. Avoid heavy sauces.

• Don't stay up too late; don't drink coffee or tea after your meal; have a glass of water for every glass of wine (or unit of alcohol) you drink.

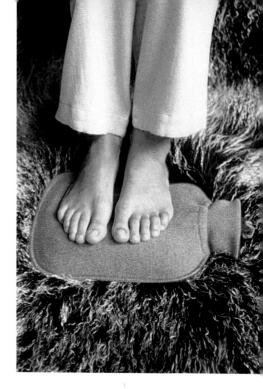

 KEY FACTS

* If you tend to 'pay for' parties with a huge hangover the morning after, learn how to prepare for them.

* Plants, homeopathy, essential oils and clay will all help you: the day before, on the day itself and the day after. Be careful about your food and alcohol intake.

37

Some yoga poses are very effective for headaches caused by stress, high blood pressure and back problems. Anyone, of any age, can practise this age-old discipline. Try it!

do 'the cat'

It's more than just physical exercise

Yoga, a product of traditional Indian medicine, is a discipline of body and mind. The poses (asanas) vary in difficulty, so everyone can manage some, at whatever level of competence. You need to be in a relaxed state of mind when performing yoga and, of course, breathing has a vital role to play. The aim is not to strive to go beyond your limits but to feel inner serenity and well-being. Regular yoga sessions increase oxygenation of the bloodstream, stimulate the body's metabolism, relieve back, neck

1

and shoulder problems, improve digestion and the cardiovascular system and calm the nerves.

Do the cat!

The cat pose is calming, relaxing and relieves the tensions that build up in the back, shoulders, neck and abdomen.
① Lie on your front, toes pointing behind you, hands flat on the ground level with your shoulders, elbows tight to your sides.
• Breathe in deeply and push up with your hands until you're on all fours.

② Breathe out and slowly sit back onto your heels.
• Keep your arms well stretched out in front of you and stay in this position for as long as possible to relax and stretch your back.

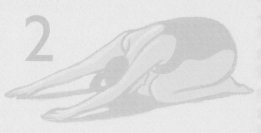

KEY FACTS

* Certain yoga poses relieve headaches caused by stress, back, neck and shoulder problems, and high blood pressure.

* The cat pose relaxes the spine.

* Regular yoga sessions should be complemented by a generally healthy lifestyle: diet, breathing and meditation.

38

plants to kill pain

Certain medicinal plants have a painkilling effect. Properly used, they are as effective as drugs, with far fewer side effects. Save chemical painkillers for emergencies only and let nature cure ordinary headaches.

More active ingredients, fewer side effects

Medicinal plants contain natural active ingredients that are copied by the pharmaceutical industry when manufacturing drugs. Manufactured drugs are often more effective and act faster, but they can be aggressive. Plants contain dozens of active elements, which is why they can be assimilated more easily and cause fewer side effects. In manufactured

● ● ● DID YOU KNOW?

> If you don't have the time or the inclination to prepare infusions and decoctions, herbal medicines are now available in new forms.

> Pharmacies and health shops sell plant essences in capsule form (containing powder, spray), phials of liquid extracts, titrated extracts (in which the active principles are standardized), macerations (plants soaked in alcohol) and so on.

drugs, on the other hand, the most effective active ingredient is isolated.

If your headaches come at regular intervals, try using herbal medicine and you'll avoid the problems that come from the regular use of painkilling and anti-inflammatory drugs. Reserve these for emergencies only and they won't lose their effectiveness.

Plants that relieve pain

• **Verbena** (Verveine), the herb of Venus: contains verbalin, which is why the plant has tonic, digestive and antispasmodic effects. Put 50g (2oz) in 1 litre ($1^3/_4$ pints) of cold water, boil for 1 minute, then leave to infuse for 10 minutes. Drink 4 cups a day between meals.

• **Meadowsweet:** salicylic acid, the basis for aspirin, was extracted from this plant. It is a very effective analgesic. Add 1 teaspoonful to a cup of boiling water and leave to infuse for 10 minutes. Drink 3 cups a day between meals.

• **Jasmine:** a wonderful way of soothing and relieving headaches due to stress. Put 20g ($^3/_4$oz) in 1 litre ($1^3/_4$ pints) of boiling water and infuse for 5 minutes. Drink 2 cupfuls a day.

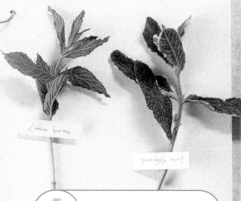

Lemon balm

pineapple mint

> Some formats are more suited to some plants than others. Check with your doctor or pharmacist and at the same ask about possible interactions with any other medication you are taking.

39

avoid acidity

Dietary imbalance and alterations in minerals in the blood may cause a number of ill effects, such as depression, tiredness, anxiety, circulation problems and headaches. To avoid them, take a careful look at what you eat.

Not too much acid, nor too little

Good health depends, among other things, on the level of acid in the blood. The body has mechanisms to keep the level within a narrow range. Practitioners of natural medicine talk of the acid-base balance. This is a rather complicated way of expressing a simple fact: the level of acidity and minerals such as potassium, sodium, magnesium and calcium inside our bodies (lymph fluid, intra- and extra-

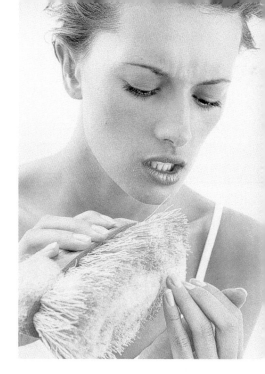

cellular fluids) depends in part on what we eat. Metabolic processes are disturbed if an imbalance lasts for too long. Over-production of stomach acid is another problem; this may be aggravated by a fatty diet and is associated with indigestion and heartburn and thus headache.

Eat more vegetables and fruit

You can easily regain the right level of acidity by eating a balanced diet. Meat is a good source of protein and red meat of iron, but it can be fatty and is in any case low in fibre. Alcohol, tea and coffee and fatty foods such as certain cuts of meat and full cream dairy products are associated with symptoms of stomach 'acidity' and can cause indigestion and heartburn, while other foods, such as egg-white, can be rather indigestible.

On the other hand, vegetables and fruit are not a good source of protein but do provide minerals such as potassium and fibre. However some fruits and vegetables, such as onions, cucumbers, tomatoes and peppers can be associated with gastric reflux and heartburn. Finally, it's worth pointing out that stress and overwork cause excess stomach acidity, as do smoking and lack of exercise.

 KEY FACTS

* Headaches are sometimes caused by excess acidity in ` the body.

* Good health depends on maintaining the correct level of acids in the blood.

* As a general rule, avoid fatty foods, alcohol and coffee and eat more vegetables and fruit.

40 stay away from smells

If pain is hammering away in your head and you're feeling nauseous, strong smells may be to blame. The only thing to do is to put distance between yourself and them.

Offensive smells Studies examining the relationship between smells and headaches have found that, even when not actually suffering, those prone to headaches have a highly developed sense of smell. However, we still don't know exactly why strong smells give some people headaches.

The only solution – flee! This, unfortunately, is best advice we can give to headache-sufferers who are bothered by strong smells. However, you may also find the following tips useful:
- Air your rooms regularly by opening the windows.
- Make sure you always have on you a handkerchief soaked in a favourite perfume, to hold to your nose if you encounter an upsetting odour.
- Spray a pleasant smelling essential oil in your home, car and office.

KEY FACTS

* Many regular headache sufferers cannot tolerate strong smells and many believe they are the cause of their problem.

* The smells most often blamed are those of perfumes, tobacco, fried food, paint and coffee.

case study

I got rid of my headaches, thanks to an elderly herbalist!

« I'm a company rep and spend a lot of time on the road. A year ago, I stopped off in a little village, as I was early for an appointment just a few miles away. I went into this very old herbalist's shop; I don't why I did, but the visit changed my life. Migraine has run in my family for several generations. I mentioned this to the lady selling the herbal medicines. When I told her that I was very shy, she exclaimed "You're suffering from emotional migraines!" She then took a packet out from behind the counter. It was a mixture of flowers and dried leaves. I was to prepare an infusion and drink about half a litre (1 pint) of it daily. Having used painkilling drugs for as long as I can remember, I was a bit sceptical of old-fashioned remedies. But I thought to myself, there's no harm in trying it. Ever since then, I carry a bottle of it around wherever I go. It may be an odd colour but it certainly works! »

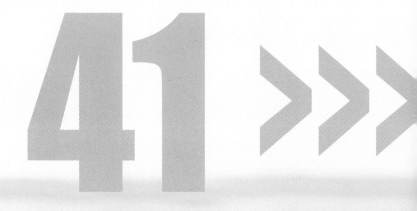

41 >>>

>> Headaches can sometimes seem an almost permanent fixture. They strike relentlessly one after another with just short periods of remission.

>>>> **If you are a chronic sufferer,** you need to discover the root cause of the trouble. Here are some possible causes, along with suggested treatments.

>>>>>> **If western medical advice doesn't solve your problems,** perhaps Chinese medicine will have some answers, and if a thermal cure doesn't interest you, maybe a therapist will suit you better.

60
TIPS

Some doctors think that chronic headaches are caused by a sudden imbalance in the autonomic nervous system. The way this system reacts depends on character, constitution and lifestyle. Make a note of your reactions: the more you understand your headaches, the better you'll be able to cure them.

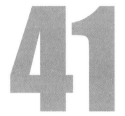

41
get to know your headaches

How it works

In the human body the autonomic nervous system controls such functions as digestion, breathing and blood circulation, over which we have no conscious control. It is made up of two parts: the sympathetic nervous system, which prepares the body for flight or fight by increasing the rate and force of the heartbeat, raising blood pressure, constricting blood vessels and diverting blood flow to the muscles, heart and brain. The parasympathetic system, however, regulates visceral activity and absorption of food. It slows the heart, opens blood vessels and reduces blood pressure, while the smooth muscle of the gut contracts to pass food along and the digestive glands release secretions to aid digestion. The system sends information to the body's organs by means of hormones. If you're in perfect health, these two parts are in harmony but humans are seldom perfectly balanced! We tend to be either energetic, spontaneous, even nervous and excitable (with a dominant sympathetic system) or thoughtful, slow and even lethargic (with a dominant parasympathetic system). Headaches can be the result of a sudden change in this delicate system.

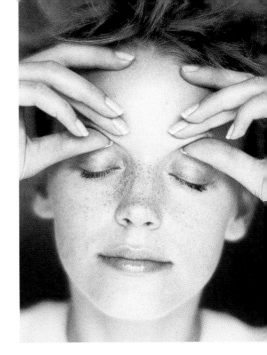

Are you a 'sympathetic' type?

If this description fits, your headaches might be caused by the widening of blood vessels in the brain. The sympathetic system orders the blood vessels to contract when necessary, whilst the parasympathetic system makes them dilate. In some people this balance is disrupted by stress, irritation, sudden hormonal change or alterations in routine. If the parasympathetic system is dominant, it brings about a sudden dilation of the blood vessels on the meninges (membranes surrounding the brain) and surface of the brain and this can give rise to a throbbing headache.

KEY FACTS

* Some headaches are caused by sudden changes in the activity of the autonomic nervous system.

* The sympathetic and parasympathetic nervous systems should be in equilibrium. Disturbances in the autonomic nervous system may trigger a dilation of blood vessels in the head and cause pain.

42

To avoid sudden changes within your autonomic nervous system, try to lead a well-regulated life. Learn to accept the kind of person you are and your head will feel much better.

know your
own rhythm

Stress and your lifestyle

Very often stress, internal or external, is at the root of the problem.
• Examples of internal stress can be a sudden fall in blood sugar levels (hypoglycaemia) or a sudden change in hormonal secretions (menstruation).
• It's much easier to deal with external forms of stress. Consider, for instance, someone in whom the parasympathetic

● ● ● DID YOU KNOW?

> When you've got a better understanding of your headaches, discuss them with the people you live with. You need their help in reshaping your routine.

> They should accept that you need these transition periods, particularly when you're first trying to adapt. Otherwise you won't succeed.

system is dominant. All week she works under stress, which boosts her sympathetic system to an unnaturally high level. When the weekend comes, she relaxes, her parasympathetic system takes over – and she gets headaches. The same thing will happen to the naturally busy 'sympathetic' person, if she winds down too much at the weekend.

Winding down without tears

To put matters right, you need above all to identify the occasions that trigger the pain: do you get headaches at the weekend or the beginning of the holidays, just before your period, when you haven't eaten for a long while or when you've had to suppress your anger?

When you've worked this out, you can take the appropriate measures. For example:

• If your headaches come at the weekend, don't suddenly change from being very busy to doing practically nothing. Be active on Saturday morning (shopping, gardening and so on) and then slow down gently.

• At the start of the holidays, spend two or three days being active but then gradually reduce the intensity of this activity during this time until you're in full relaxation mode.

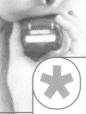

> If you force yourself to do what other people want in order to please them, your autonomic nervous system will rush into action again … with the usual results.

43

a tonic for your type

Some plants can regulate this delicate balance. If you're predominantly a parasympathetic type, boost your sympathetic side with extracts of dandelion, blackcurrant, thyme, butcher's broom and hyssop.

The parasympathetic type

You're rather introverted and don't express your feelings very easily. You're reflective, sometimes almost withdrawn, or at least you seem to be. You're capable of brooding alone over a problem and, because you won't share it with anyone, of getting very gloomy, even depressed about it. Actually, under your reserved demeanour, you're highly emotional but you just hide it well. You need

● ● ● DID YOU KNOW?

> Blackcurrant is very good for stimulating the sympathetic system of predominantly parasympathetic people. The berries can be eaten and the leaves used to make infusions (use one tablespoonful per cup and leave to infuse for 10 minutes).

> Blackcurrant is particularly rich in vitamin C, which explains its tonic action. You can also make blackcurrant wine or liqueur (consume in moderation!).

regularity and routine. You're a marathon runner, not a sprinter. You don't feel very comfortable in groups.

The plants you need

If you're predominantly a parasympathetic type, you need plants that will strengthen your sympathetic nervous system.

- **Dandelion:** you can take in salads or as a decoction. To make a decoction, soak 30g (1¼oz) of leaves and roots in a litre (1¾pints) of cold water for 2 hours then heat gently. As soon as the water boils, remove it from the heat. Drink 3 cups a day before meals.
- **Thyme:** season your food with it or make a herbal tea. Add 30g (1¼oz) to a litre (1¾pints) of boiling water, cover and leave to infuse for 10 minutes. Carefully collect the steam that condenses on the lid, as it contains the volatile active elements. Drink 3 cups a day.
- **Butcher's broom:** put 5g (¼oz) in 500ml (17fl oz) of water, boil for 4 minutes, then allow to infuse for 10 minutes. Drink throughout the day. Do not top up the herb.
- **Hyssop:** put 1 tablespoonful in 500ml (17fl oz) of boiling water and infuse for 10 minutes. Drink throughout the course of the day. Hyssop should not be given to children.

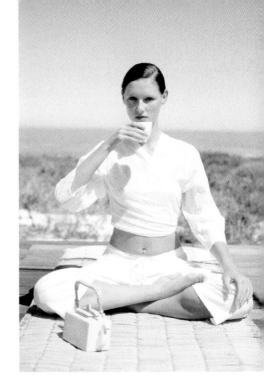

KEY FACTS

* Parasympathetic people find it difficult to express their emotions.

* Plants that can help are thyme, hyssop, butcher's broom and dandelion.

* Blackcurrant is also effective and is very rich in vitamin C.

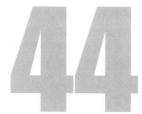

plants to calm and relax you

Emotional, fiery people whose nervous system is predominantly sympathetic need help to calm down and relax. These plants can provide gentle, natural help: German camomile, nettle, fumitory, mint and bitter orange.

The sympathetic type

The adjective has become a part of everyday language. 'Sympathetic' people expresses their feelings. They communicate readily and are very much at ease in company. This spontaneity, however, hides an anxiety deeper than you might think. A spontaneous, outgoing manner uses up a lot of the adrenaline secreted in times of stress. Sympathetic people may be hyperactive but their efforts are inconsistent. They like intense activity interspersed with periods of rest.

● ● ● DID YOU KNOW?

> The flowers, peel and leaves of the bitter orange are all used in herbal medicine.

> Neroli (orange blossom) essential oil is extracted from the flowers. Both the flowers and the leaves are sedative and antispasmodic, which is why they can help 'sympathetic' people to relax.

The plants you need

If you recognize yourself in that description, try the following plants.

• **German camomile:** add 2 tablespoonfuls to 500ml (17fl oz) of boiling water and leave to infuse for 10 minutes. After drinking this herbal tea, you should rest for a little while in a darkened room.

• **Nettle:** both species of nettle (Common and Small) have similar qualities. Infuse 25g (1oz) of the plant in 500ml (17fl oz) of boiling water for 15 minutes. Drink one cup per day.

• **Fumitory:** infuse 20g (³/₄oz) in 500ml (17fl oz) of boiling water for 10 minutes. Drink one cup every day for a week. After that, stop for at least 10 days before repeating.

• **Mint:** infuse 5g (¹/₄oz) of mint leaves in 250ml (8fl oz) of boiling water for 10 minutes. Drink a cup of the infusion before going to bed.

> Infuse a teaspoonful of dried leaves in a cup of boiling water for 10 minutes. You can also add 5 drops of neroli essential oil mixed with bubble bath to your bath on a regular basis.

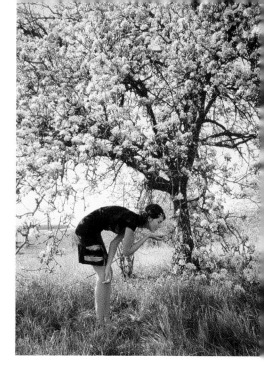

KEY FACTS

＊ 'Sympathetic' people are extroverted, open and at ease in the company of others.

＊ However they can also be anxious and inconsistent in their efforts.

＊ The plants they should take are German camomile, nettle, mint, fumitory and bitter orange.

45

avoid arguments

Some people suffer from headaches when they get annoyed. If you're one of them, you can't always expect those you live with to keep quiet and put up with all your whims. You've got to learn to compromise.

When two become one

In a couple, one person often has a dominant sympathetic nervous system and the other a dominant parasympathetic system. This often reflects our natural tendency to look for a complementary difference in our partner, whether in love or friendship. There's no problem if each allows the other some time to be him/herself but if one of the couple dominates, the other has to put up with it and is forced to suppress his/her inner nature. The autonomic nervous system is affected by the distortion and eventually reacts.

Accept your partner but don't suppress yourself

When a sympathetic type lives with a parasympathetic one, he/she sometimes feels the need to slow down to please the other person. If this happens too often, the parasympathetic system reacts and headaches can be the result. The same thing happens if a parasympathetic person forces him/herself to be excessively active and energetic.

To avoid these difficult outcomes, each partner should accept the other's nature without sacrificing their own. This is the best way to avoid the confrontations, tensions and conflicts that often cause violent headaches in those who are susceptible to them.

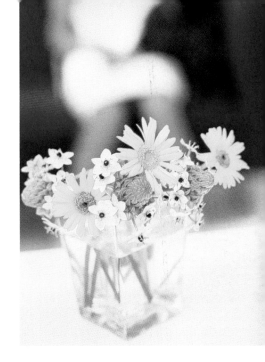

> If you are susceptible to headaches, consider whether your children are sympathetic or parasympathetic. Teach them to accept themselves for what they are without suppressing their nature or dominating that of others. It's vital to their adult welfare.

 KEY FACTS

* Couples (friends, husband and wife, etc.) often complement each other: one sympathetic and one parasympathetic person.

* If this is the case, each person must accept it and allow their partner time to be him/herself. If not, the frustration felt by the one who is always giving way is likely to cause headaches.

46

come to terms with your emotions

Some headaches are caused by psychological factors like the inability to manage emotions. It may be time to learn to manage this aspect of your self.

We do not see ourselves ...

Many people are overcome by their emotions because they do not know or like themselves well enough. An unkind remark or some doubt expressed makes them see red, their heart beats faster, they are completely thrown. This inner tension can lead to a painful headache. Whether you fly into a temper or are unable to express your displeasure, whether you keep silent or burst into a long tirade, the essential thing is to learn to understand, accept and express yourself. The more you try to suppress a strong, recurrent emotion, the more it will harden inside you and look for a way out against your will. On the other hand, if you acknowledge the emotion, it will gradually fade away.

… as we really are

There are several psycho-emotional techniques that can help your self-confidence. An approach such as that of Gestalt therapy, for example, leads to an awareness of a crucial fact: our perception of ourselves and the world around us does not consist merely of what we feel or see on the surface. This form of therapy relates our perception to its psychological and physical environment. We do not perceive objectively. We

create our own reality, because our senses allow us to see only what suits us at the time. Gestalt therapy seeks to make us aware of our 'avoidance mechanisms', so we can achieve a broader and more tolerant understanding of those around us and of ourselves.

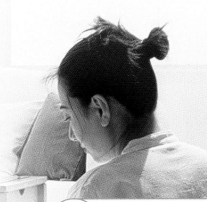

> In this way, the patient is led to express a feeling, study an attitude or plumb an emotion and to achieve greater self-esteem.

KEY FACTS

* Emotions can be overwhelming if we do not know or like ourselves well enough. This feeling of being overwhelmed can give rise to headaches.

* Psycho-emotional techniques like Gestalt therapy can help us to be more tolerant and to accept ourselves more readily.

47

steer clear of conflict

Conflict is another factor that disturbs your inner balance and so causes headaches. Conflicts always result from misunderstandings and misunderstandings occur when there has been a failure in communication. Transactional analysis seeks to repair these breakdowns.

The theory

Transactional analysis is an accessible method of understanding how each individual functions, both within him/herself and with others. Learning to analyse the interplay or 'transactions' between ourselves and other people enables us to understand how we handle our life. Transactional analysis is based upon a novel conception of what happens to us

● ● ● DID YOU KNOW?

> In the 1960s, Eric Berne developed transactional analysis. One of the foundations of his theory is the concept of human personality being made up of three 'ego states': the child, the parent and the adult. The parent establishes the rules; the adult thinks rationally and takes the decisions; the child feels and reacts. These three states interact and form the basis from which we interact with others. They need to be in equilibrium for inner harmony. In western society

in life: nothing, or almost nothing, really happens 'by chance'. It is as if we have been programmed by education, culture, habits and experiences. Automatically and without thinking, we behave as we have been programmed and this causes conflicts in ourseleves that eventually lead to headaches.

The practice

The therapy consists of discovering the nature of your 'transactions' with other people – which part of you is communicating? The part that has learnt, the part that thinks or the part that feels? Transactional analysis reveals the different scenarios we regularly repeat within ourselves and in our relationships with others. A lasting change is achieved when the person concerned understands and feels what makes him or her behave as

he or she does and, with the therapist's help and encouragement, acquires the ability to express the emotions associated with this behaviour.

it is usually the child that is suppressed, submissive, dormant. Consequently, we become individuals governed only by our adult and parent states: in other words, reasonable, responsible, respectable but also sad, tired and ... suffering from headaches.

KEY FACTS

* Continual conflict causes headaches in those who are susceptible.

* Learning to communicate better avoids unnecessary conflicts.

* This is what transactional analysis sets out to achieve.

48

Some recurrent headaches are due to hormonal changes. They particularly affect women just before their periods or during the menopause. Analysing and regulating these hormones can cure this type of headache.

check out your hormones

Relationships, pleasure and the enjoyment of life

Everyone, male or female, is influenced from earliest childhood to the end of life by the continual interplay of hormones. They give us energy, sensations of excitement and the desire to procreate. They can make existence joyful, relationships deeply satisfying and our outlook bright and optimistic. However, when their levels drop, our mood darkens and our

● ● ●   DID YOU KNOW?

> Nowadays vegetable hormones from plants such as soya and yam can be used to correct female hormonal imbalances in a natural way.

> The first contains phyto-oestrogen and the second a substance that produces progesterone. The body can use these natural substances to make up for what it lacks.

relationships, including our sex life, suffer. Sudden variations in the secretion of hormones can sometimes be very stressful and give rise to headaches. Women are the most affected, because their hormones are linked to regular cycles so that there is a much greater risk of an imbalance.

Premenstrual syndrome and the menopause

The female cycle is normally like the lunar month, that is to say, it is repeated every 28 days. During the first half of the cycle, the body secretes mainly oestrogens to prepare for ovulation. Then it begins to secrete progesterone to stimulate the formation of the placenta in readiness for a possible embryo. If no egg is fertilized, menstruation removes all this unwanted tissue and the body prepares to begin all over again. Some women find these hormonal variations

difficult to cope with. Perhaps they happen too suddenly or there is too little or too much of one of the hormones. These factors can make the days just before periods very painful: fluid retention, hot flushes, mood swings and headaches can occur. These problems become increasingly serious with the onset of the menopause. They can, however, be solved by boosting the hormones at different times in the cycle. Sometimes simply taking the combined oral contraceptive pill may be enough to control premenstrual syndrome but sometimes more detailed advice from a specialist is helpful.

> Because natural treatments contain less active substance they may be more easily tolerated than chemical hormonal substitutes but somewhat less effective.

KEY FACTS

* Sudden variations in the hormone levels can create internal stress and therefore cause headaches.

* This is particularly so in the case of women around menstruation, puberty or the menopause.

* Your doctor may be able to prescribe medication for you and give you advice about further investigations.

49

therapy may help

Some people end up organizing their whole life around their headaches. They find that they bring certain advantages they're reluctant to give up. That's when therapy can help.

The body sends messages

Nothing that happens to your body is entirely without some connection with your mind. Some headaches are directly due to accumulated psychological tension. A visit to a psychotherapist will give you an opportunity to talk about it and can help you decipher your body's messages. Difficulty in accepting certain thoughts, ideas, feelings, pressures or

● ● ● DID YOU KNOW?

> A psychologist is not necessarily a therapist. With a degree in psychology and further clinical training, s/he analyses and diagnoses problems and, if necessary, refers you to a specialist. Treatments include counselling, cognitive therapy for depression and behavioural modification to treat phobias.

> Therapists offer 'talking treatments' for psychological problems. Although the origin of therapy probably lies with Freud, there are now many types of therapists with a wide range of training. Before choosing, learn about a therapist's approach and training.

frustrations, career problems or family conflict may cause stress which is then expressed as headache – a tight band of pain around the head or a throbbing headache. This is what is known as tension headache.

However, it doesn't do to oversimplify things: each body has its own way of expressing itself according to the experiences of the individual to whom it belongs!

Illuminating the depths

Well-conducted psychotherapy can lead to an insight into why you are getting headaches in the first place. For example, the pain might have certain advantages. For some people, it's a way of escaping from onerous responsibilities or of gaining more attention than they would normally get. The conscious desire to be free of headaches clashes with the unconscious wish to keep them because of the benefits they bring. By talking about the problem, it may be possible to untangle this intimate and complex web and see things more clearly. This can sometimes be enough to stop the headaches when they become psychologically unnecessary.

> A psychoanalyst is a more highly trained therapist who tends to offer intensive treatments of several sessions a week for some years. Classically s/he's the one who asks you to lie down on a couch and talk.
> Only a psychiatrist is also a trained doctor as well: s/he deals with very serious cases of mental disturbance and tends to use drug treatments.

KEY FACTS

* Headaches may be the body's way of expressing difficulty in accepting certain thoughts, ideas or feelings.

* Sometimes headaches can bring advantages that, unconsciously, we don't want to give up.

* Once we understand our tangled motivations, we can rid ourselves of pointless pain.

50 you're magnetic!

Magnets can be used to relax muscles and relieve pain. This is an effective treatment for headaches caused by muscular and bone problems.

An age-old technique Some headaches, such as Arnold's neuralgias, are caused by damage to the nerves or to the vertebrae in the neck, or by muscular spasms. Magnetotherapy is a technique that involves placing small magnets on the painful areas. It doesn't take long for the spasms, inflammation and pain to disappear. The technique is an age-old remedy and is mentioned in both ancient Chinese and Hindu texts that date back thousands of years BCE.

How does it work? Magnets can relieve pain through bio-magnetism, in other words, the sensitivity that all living matter has to the earth's magnetic field. It is thought that we possess special magnetic receptors in our fingertips, at the back of the neck and also in the hips, knees and sinuses. Basically, a magnet has analgesic qualities: its north pole is relaxing, whilst its south pole has a painkilling and anti-inflammatory effect.

● ● ● DID YOU KNOW?

> You can buy magnets at your pharmacy. Just simply place them on the pain points. In about 80% of cases the pain goes away. There are specialist therapists who can effectively place the magnets on the appropriate nerve fibres well away from the actual pain.

KEY FACTS

* Magnetotherapy involves placing little magnets on the painful area.

* It can be an effective way of relieving some headaches.

51 look after your teeth

The body can react adversely to poorly aligned or uneven teeth or if fillings are badly done or cracked, with underlying pulp infection. Sometimes these factors can cause intense headaches, although the exact reason for this remains a mystery. Tooth grinding at night may also give rise to headaches.

It's something you can easily fail to notice When teeth are badly positioned, the alignment of the jaw itself may be slightly altered. This can distort its movements when you are chewing and the problem can have repercussions on the neck muscles. From there the pain can descend as far as the lumbar vertebrae but it's more frequently felt in the back of the head, the temples or the forehead.

Check with your dentist You shouldn't hesitate to visit the dentist if you suffer from recurrent headaches and suspect that your teeth may be behind them. It's preferable to choose a specialist in orthodontics. He will be able to tell if your teeth and jaw are badly aligned when you chew and, if so, which teeth are to blame.

● ● ● DID YOU KNOW?

> Tooth-grinding may be responsible for your headaches.
> You may not even be aware that you grind your teeth. Many people actually grind their teeth in their sleep.

KEY FACTS

* Badly aligned or uneven teeth can cause muscular tension that leads to violent headaches.

* Consult a dentist, preferably an orthodontist. He will be able to tell if your teeth are to blame.

* Have your fillings checked regularly.

52

back to
the bones

The human body is a very precise mechanism. Its skeletal structure is capable of making minute adjustments when necessary. However, if this structure is forced to maintain an awkward position for too long or undergoes a series of impacts, it is liable to 'protest' and headaches can be the result.

Try an osteopath

It may seem odd to consult a specialist in bones, joints and muscles to find a cure for headaches, but it's not as strange as it seems. Arthritis in the neck vertebrae can cause headaches that start at the back of the head and move forward across the skull. Osteopathy is based on the concept that the skeleton and muscles constantly interact with all the other bodily systems. An osteopath looks for tiny anomalies in the muscular-skeletal system and cures them by means of gentle but firm manipulations. Cranial osteopathy concentrates on tiny, imperceptible movements of the skull. When the skull is 'articulated' correctly, there is an even flow of spinal fluid. The body's capacity for self-healing, for seeking balance and health, does the rest.

Referred pain

Painful reactions can sometimes make themselves felt a long way from the origin of the problem. When the body has to cope with a joint in an awkward position, it begins by making an adjustment. Initially, this is easily done and no discomfort is felt. However the muscles that have to adjust eventually grow tired and inflamed. This is why you can sometimes have a backache because your knee is in an uncomfortable position or a headache because of a problem in your neck.

> This is why a successful course of osteopathy can make you feel great again if you've been feeling depressed.

KEY FACTS

* Headaches are sometimes caused by an uncomfortably positioned bone or joint in another part of the body.

* Osteopathy can correct these malfunctions and relieve the pain.

* Cranial osteopathy concentrates entirely on miniscule and imperceptible adjustments of the bones in the skull.

53

try trace elements

Maybe your headaches are simply caused by a lack of trace elements? These minerals are present in tiny quantities in the body and yet play an essential role as the catalyst in countless biochemical reactions vital to life.

'Trace' equals small, very small!

Trace elements are present in the body in such tiny quantities that for a long time they were considered to be a sort of waste material until around 1890, when it was realized that they were indispensable to life. Without them a number of biochemical reactions would take place with great difficulty, if at all. A shortage of trace elements can cause rheumatism, insomnia, tiredness and, of course, headaches.

Trace elements that may help

• **Magnesium:** thought to play an essential part in the working of the central nervous system, being necessary for the passage of nerve impulses between the brain cells. It also helps those whose headaches are caused by high blood pressure.

• **Manganese:** a trace element that may help to suppress allergies, is sometimes a very effective means of getting rid of very stubborn headaches. Combined with cobalt it could relieve headaches due to hormonal imbalances caused by the menopause.

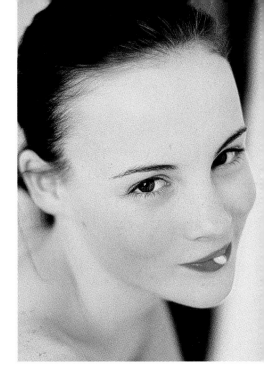

> A sample of blood or, more effectively, of hair, will indicate whether you are deficient in trace elements or not. Do note that in the UK such tests are not available on the NHS.

  KEY FACTS

* Headaches can sometimes be due to a shortage of trace elements.

* These minerals are present in the body in tiny amounts but play an indispensable part in the millions of biochemical reactions essential for the maintenance of life.

54 put some colour in your life

Did you know that colours can relieve pain, particularly headaches? If chosen correctly, coloured beams of light penetrate the body and bring it relief. Try chromotherapy!

> A 1977 study undertaken at Lille University, in France, proved that certain bacteria die if they are exposed to blue or violet light, while red light kills the strepto- coccus and staphylococcus bacteria plus the diphtheria bacterium.

> It is also known that cucumbers cultivated under a red light grow larger than ones that aren't, whilst a blue light increases the vitamin C content of the leaves.

Electromagnetic rays

Colours and light influence mood: blue tends to have a calming effect and red a stimulating one. These responses are not simply psychological. Colours are, in fact, electromagnetic rays of different wavelengths. The eye receives them and the brain translates them into sensations of colour. As for the body, it absorbs and reacts to them. For example, newborn babies suffering from jaundice are put under blue lamps as this wavelength breaks down the bilirubin responsible for the illness, and the ultra-violet rays in sunlight helps the skin manufacture vitamin D for strong healthy bones. Chromotherapy works for headaches too: treatment is by means of appropriately chosen coloured lights.

Colours release energy

To relieve pain, coloured rays of light are directed at acupuncture points. The therapist chooses the colour according to the form of energy it releases. For instance, red gives off a hot energy, green a dry energy and orange a cold energy. The therapist then selects the acupuncture point according to the principles of energy flow used in traditional Chinese medicine, and directs a very fine beam from a fibre-optic light onto this area. The treatment doesn't take very long (generally about ten minutes) and two or three sessions are usually enough for positive effects to be observed. Beams of coloured light are very effective in curing inflammatory illnesses and some headaches come into this category.

KEY FACTS

* Chromotherapy treats headaches by directing beams of coloured light onto specific acupuncture points.

* The points and colours are chosen according to the effect desired.

* A session lasts about ten minutes and positive results can be observed after two or three sessions.

> Finally, fish eggs hatch more or less quickly according to the quality of light that reaches them, proving that light definitely has an effect on living creatures.

treat yourself
to a spa cure

All spa waters, whether hot or cold, whether from a source deep within the earth or on the surface, have medicinal qualities: some contain sulphur, some sulphate, some magnesium and some greater or lesser quantities of other minerals. Some of the waters are very useful for curing headaches.

Water, water everywhere

Spa towns such as Vittel and Vichy in France specialize in providing treatment for headaches. This is largely due to the special qualities of their waters. Vittel water is particularly rich in magnesium, a mineral that is vital to the functioning of the brain and central nervous system.

In general, cold waters containing metallic trace elements are diuretic and waters with a calcium sulphate content

● ● ● DID YOU KNOW?

> A full thermal cure lasts for three weeks and is taken under medical supervision. Shorter courses of treatment to help get you back into good shape are available.

> Treatments offered include baths, showers, wraps, compresses, poultices, colonic irrigation, power showers and massage. Of course, you can also drink the water, inhale it or gargle with it.

cleanse the liver, whilst carbonic waters are sedative and help the digestive system to function properly.

Taking stock of yourself

But there's more to a thermal cure than just the waters. When you're a chronic headache sufferer, the original cause of the illness gets mixed up with a lot of other factors over the years. A thermal cure is an opportunity to take stock, to understand yourself better.

That's why the facilities at spas often include ancillary services. At Vichy, a team of psychologists and psychotherapists is available for consultation if your headaches have a psychological aspect. At Vittel, a dentist is on hand to check whether headaches are due to problems with the patient's 'bite'. Other centres offer sophrology or shiatsu sessions. You should research your nearest spa and the facilities it offers.

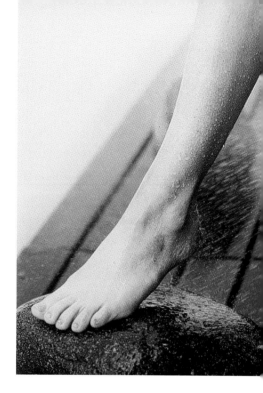

> Many thalassotherapy centres also offer 'dry treatments' such as massage, relaxation, relaxation therapy and energy-flow medicine.

 KEY FACTS

* Because the characteristics of their waters differ, spas specialize in different illnesses.

* Some spas offer treatments specially targeted at curing headaches.

* Ancillary services are usually available, too.

56 essential oils

Essential oils are the concentrated extracts of medicinal plants. Sometimes a simple massage with essential oils is all it takes to relieve a headache.

Natural active ingredients An essential oil is usually extracted from the plant by steam distillation. Its active essences are highly concentrated. For example, it takes 5,000kg (5 tons) of rosebuds to produce 1kg (2lb) of rose essential oil. Essential oils have many beneficial effects, including anti-inflammatory, invigorating, healing or stimulating, to mention just a few of them.

Essential oils and headaches The essential oils of lavender (*Lavandula officinalis*) and peppermint (*Mentha piperita*) are very effective against headaches: put three drops on your fingertips and massage your temples or the back of your neck, making small, circular motions.
You might also try helichrysum (*H. angustifolia*) essential oil. It's also known as boxer's oil, because it relieves pains caused by a blow – and headaches can feel just like that!

KEY FACTS

* Essential oils are concentrated extracts of plants that have medicinal properties.

* Some of them are particularly effective in soothing painful headaches.

* They are for external use only, unless prescribed otherwise by a doctor.

●●● D I D   Y O U   K N O W ?

> Because essential oils are very concentrated, they can sometimes be toxic if swallowed. Unless you are taking them under medical supervision, make sure that you use them only for massage, in a diffuser or diluted in your bath water.

57 acupuncture may be the answer

It's the branch of Chinese medicine we're most familiar with in the Western world. An acupuncturist clears energy blockages with the use of needles and headaches can be gone in a trice!

Vital energy on command Every living thing needs vital energy. It circulates along internal channels, or meridians, fuelling all our organs. Sometimes this energy gets blocked, causing headaches, among other problems. To make the pain disappear, the blockage needs to be cleared.

Too much Yin or too much Yang? Energy is made up of two opposing principles, the Yin and the Yang, which must always remain in balance. The first is characteristically cold, fluid, wet, slow, sombre, whilst the second is hot, solid, dry, quick and lively. In order to know where to insert the needles, the acupuncturist seeks to discover the origin of the given problem: in which zone is the energy blocked? Which organ is suffering from a shortage or excess of energy? Is there too much Yin or too much Yang?

KEY FACTS

* Acupuncture involves balancing the body's flow of vital energy.

* It effective in treating headaches.

* The needles are sterile and used only once.

58

eat Chinese

Chinese medicine uses many other therapies, including diet. You can cure headaches by eating in accordance with the strict rules of energy flow.

The heart, summertime and fire

According to Chinese medicine, headaches are caused by a disruption of the energy flow within the heart meridian. Each of the five main organs of the body is linked with a symbolic element and a season. The heart is linked with fire and the summer. Therefore, if you are prone to headaches, you need to pay particular attention to what you eat in the summer.

● ● ● DID YOU KNOW?

> An excess of Yang in the heart meridian can also sometimes cause headaches of a very different kind: this type of pain is more sporadic, violent and short-lived.

> It explodes like an outburst of anger and then dies down as rapidly as it came.

The energy in the heart meridian is also responsible for the condition of the blood vessels as well as that of the blood itself. It is not surprising, therefore, that headaches are often caused by circulation problems.

Food for the heart

According to the Chinese view, everything you eat affects the energy flow: some foods are Yin, others are Yang; some are linked with the heart, others with the liver or the kidneys.

Chronic headaches are usually the result of a lack of energy – an excess of Yin – in the heart meridian. Foods that improve the circulation of energy in this meridian have a bitter, stimulating flavour (mutton, wheat, apricots, shallots and dandelions, for instance). Coffee also tastes bitter and headache sufferers don't need

telling that a good strong cup of coffee can sometimes make an attack go away. You shouldn't rely too often on this method though, because too much caffeine causes other problems, which might well make the remedy more harmful than the original malady.

> To relieve this type of headache, you need to cut out all sharp-tasting food.

KEY FACTS

* Chinese medicine advocates choosing foods according to their effects on the energy flow.

* Headaches often result from an excess of energy in the heart meridian.

* Foods that have a sharp or bitter taste often relieve headaches: mutton, apricots, shallots, dandelions and wheat, for example.

59

the Yin and Yang of plants

Medicinal herbs form another essential plank of Chinese medicine. It is believed that they, too, can regulate disorders in the energy flow, provided they are chosen according to certain principles ...

Western plants selected according to Chinese principles

The Chinese classify their medicinal plants according to their flavour and their effects on the energy flow. Some are Yin, others Yang. As with food, they are all linked to a symbolic element and one of the five main bodily organs.

> To follow a genuine course of Chinese medicine, it's best to consult a specialist who will be able to discover the exact causes of your headaches.

> Causes can vary from person to person. To complement a herbal treatment, you may be advised to go on a diet and do some Qi Gong exercises.

To treat headaches, Yang plants linked with the heart should be chosen, because they restore circulation in this meridian. However, there's no need to go to Beijing to get your plants. A team of French researchers has classified western medicinal herbs according to the criteria of Chinese medicine. You can, therefore, cure your headaches with easily available plants that conform to Chinese principles of energy.

Plants that cure headaches

Some plants should be taken as a herbal tea and others used as an essential oil.
• Use any of the following to make a herbal tea or take in capsule form: common yarrow, motherwort, angelica, wild rose, madder, fleabane, white pimpernel, red cinchona.

• Use the essential oils of the following plants (mixed with a carrier oil) for massage: angelica, bitter orange (neroli), lavender, damask rose, clary sage.

KEY FACTS

∗ Chinese medicinal plants are classified according to their flavour and effect on the body's energy flow.

∗ Western plants have been classified using the same criteria.

∗ You can use western plants to follow a course of herbal treatment that adheres to the Chinese principles of good energy flow.

> Chinese herbal remedies are unregulated in some countries. It's important to choose a reputable practitioner.

60 be careful with painkillers

Drugs are sometimes necessary to relieve the pain of some migraine attacks or persistent headaches. There are many different kinds.

For tension headaches or mild migraine a simple painkiller such as paracetamol is best and has fewest side effects. Aspirin and ibuprofen are also effective but can cause upset stomachs, bleeding from the gut or even aggravate asthma in some people. Sometimes paracetamol is combined with other drugs, such as codeine, caffeine or antihistamines, and there are also specific drugs for migraine called 'triptans' that act on serotonin receptors. For regular and persistent headaches, preventive drugs are available, such as low doses of a tricylic antidepressant or beta-blockers. These are available only on prescription and you should always discuss your symptoms with your doctor.

Never use more than you need There are very strict rules for how many triptans you can take (e.g. no more than two doses in 24 hrs). Keep them for emergencies as they become less effective if taken often and some can harm the digestive system. Never exceed the prescribed dose.

KEY FACTS

* Analgesic and anti-inflammatory drugs are often prescribed to treat headaches.

* Painkillers should be used very carefully, because they can cause side effects. Never exceed the prescribed dose.

case study

I worked out my own treatment programme

« Initially I took the usual painkillers prescribed by the doctor to try to cure my headaches,' Jeanette recalls. 'When one stopped being effective, I tried another. When I got to the twenty-third, I gave up! I realized this hunt for the miracle drug was getting me nowhere. Now I've worked out a method that involves several different approaches: I've four or five prescription painkillers that I know I can rely on but to these I've added some homeopathic medicines plus osteopathy, acupuncture and even massage sessions. Even though massage may seem to have nothing to do with migraines, I think a good, relaxing massage does me nothing but good. »

useful addresses

» Acupuncture

British Acupuncture Council
63 Jeddo Road
London W12 9HQ
tel: 020 8735 0400
www.acupuncture.org.uk

**British Medical
Acupuncture Society**
12 Marbury House
Higher Whitley, Warrington
Cheshire WA4 4QW.
tel: 01925 730727

**Australian Acupuncture
and Chinese Medicine
Association**
PO Box 5142
West End, Queensland 4101
Australia
www.acupuncture.org.au

» Homeopathy

**British Homeopathic
Association**
Hahnemann House
29 Park Street West
Luton LU1 3BE
tel: 0870 444 3950

The Society of Homeopaths
4a Artizan Road
Northampton NN1 4HU
tel: 01604 621400

**Australian Homeopathic
Association**
PO Box 430, Hastings
Victoria 3915, Australia
www.homeopathyoz.org

» Herbal medicine

**British Herbal Medicine
Association**
Sun House, Church Street
Stroud, Gloucester GL5 1JL
tel: 01453 751389

**National Institute
of Medical Herbalists**
56 Longbrook Street
Exeter, Devon EX4 6AH
tel: 01392 426022

» Massage

**British Massage Therapy
Council**
www.bmtc.co.uk

**Association of British
Massage Therapists**
42 Catharine Street
Cambridge CB1 3AW
tel: 01223 240 815

European Institute of Massage
42 Moreton Street
London SW1V 2PB
tel: 020 7931 9862

» Qi Gong

**Qi Gong Association
of America**
PO Box 252
Lakeland, MN, USA
email: info@nqa.org

**World Natural Medicine
Foundation**
College of Medical Qi Gong
9904 106 Street,
Edmonton AB T5K IC4
Canada

» Relaxation therapy

British Autogenic Society
The Royal London
Homoeopathic Hospital
Greenwell Street
London W1W 5BP

**British Complementary
Medicine Association**
PO Box 5122
Bournemouth BH8 0WG
tel: 0845 345 5977

» Yoga

The British Wheel of Yoga
25 Jermyn Street
Sleaford, Lincs NG34 7RU
tel: 01529 306 851
www.bwy.org.uk

index

acknowledgements

Cover: J. Toy/Stone; p. 8-9: B. Yee/Photonica; p. 10-11: P. Viant/Pix; p. 13: T. Shinoda/Photonica; p. 15: R. Wright/Stone; p. 17, 19, 22, 67, 73, 80-81, 97, 98-99, 100-101, 104-105, 112: Neo Vision/Photonica; p. 21: A. Parker/Option Photo; p. 25: A. Peisl/Zefa; p. 29: © Akiko Ida; p. 32-33: J. McBride/Stone; p. 35: G. Girardot/Marie Claire; p. 36-37: A. Peisl/Zefa; p. 45: J. Sebag/Stock Image; p. 48-49: David Paul Productions/Image Bank; p. 51: A. Parker/Option photo; p. 53: © Photothéque Hachette; p. 58: T. Haus/Marie Claire; p. 61: M. Gravenor/Stone; p. 75: B. Anderson/Marie Claire; p. 77: Cora/Marie Claire; p. 83: H. Brehm/Marie-Claire; p. 87: A. Wyant/Stone; p. 89: S. Lancrenon/Marie Claire; p. 90-91: P. Pacifica/Image Bank; p. 93: A. Peisl/Zefa; p. 95: N. La Ganza/Stock Image; p. 109: H. Scheibe/Zefa; p. 111: F. Deconick/Marie Claire; p. 115: M. Montezin/Marie Claire; p. 118-119, 120-121: D.R.

Illustrations: Marianne Maury Kaufmann pages 42-43, 62-63, 64, 68, 78-79; Anne Cinquanta pages 56-57.

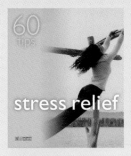

stress relief

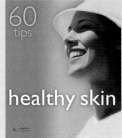

healthy skin

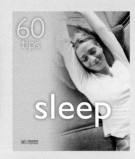

sleep

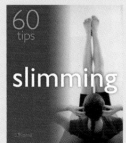

slimming

The 60 Tips
collection
All the keys,
all the tips
and all the
answers to
your health
questions

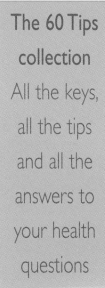

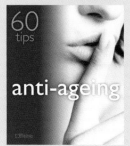

anti-ageing

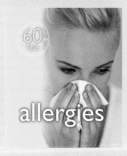

allergies

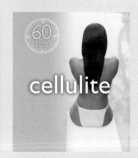

cellulite

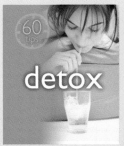

detox

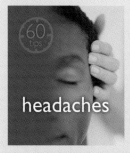

headaches

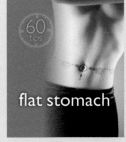

flat stomach

Editorial director: Caroline Rolland

Editorial assistant: Marine Barbier

Graphic design and layout: G & C MOI

Final checking: Marie-Claire Seewald

Illustrations: Alexandra Bentz

Production: Felicity O'Connor

Translation: JMS Books LLP

A CIP catalogue for this book is available from the British Library

ISBN-13: 978-1-84430-089-1

ISBN-10: 1-84430-089-7

Printed in Singapore by Tien Wah Press